Artificial Intelligence in Oncology Drug Discovery and Development

Edited by John W. Cassidy and Belle Taylor

Published in London, United Kingdom

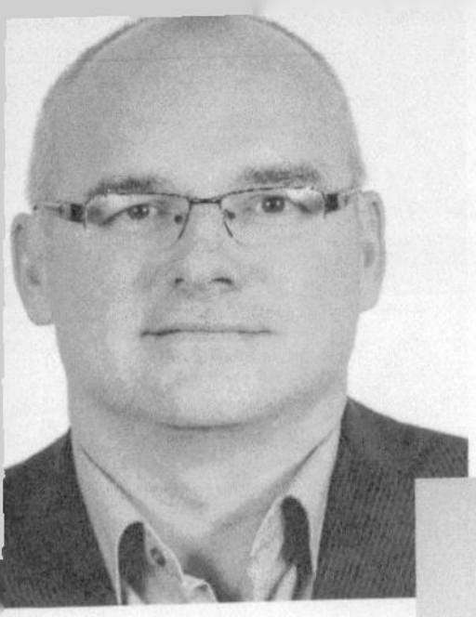
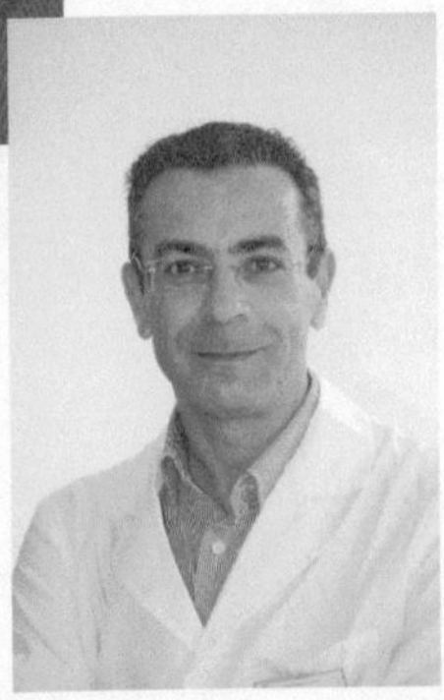
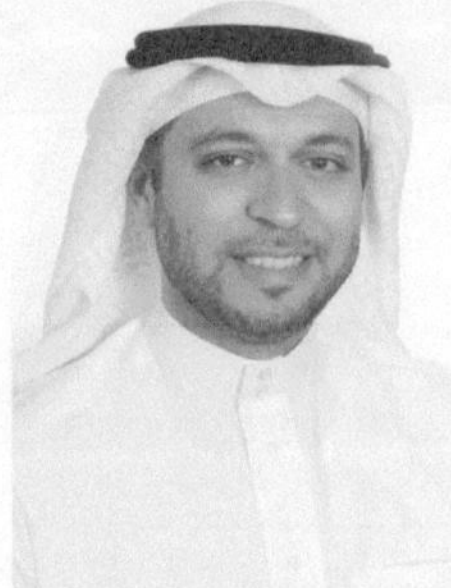
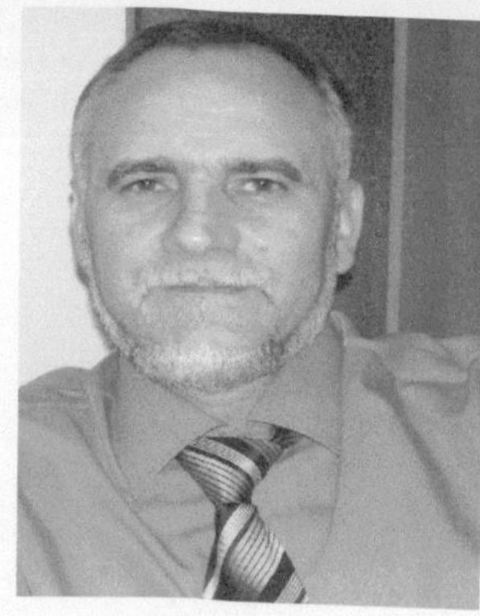
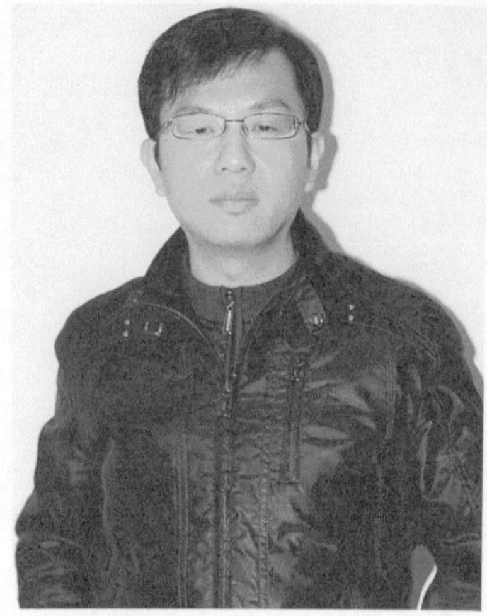
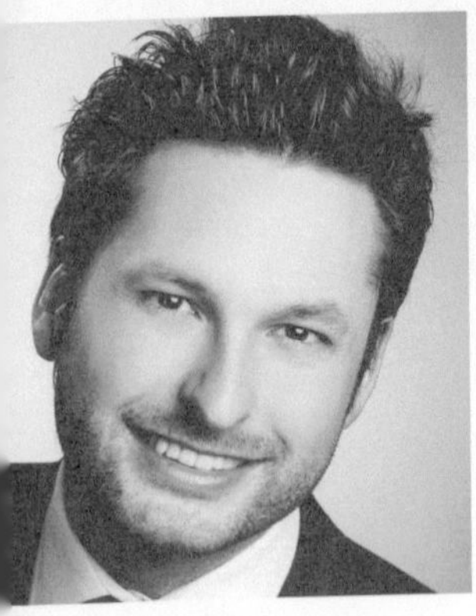
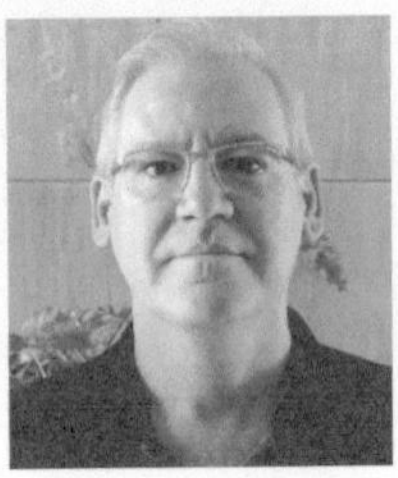

IntechOpen

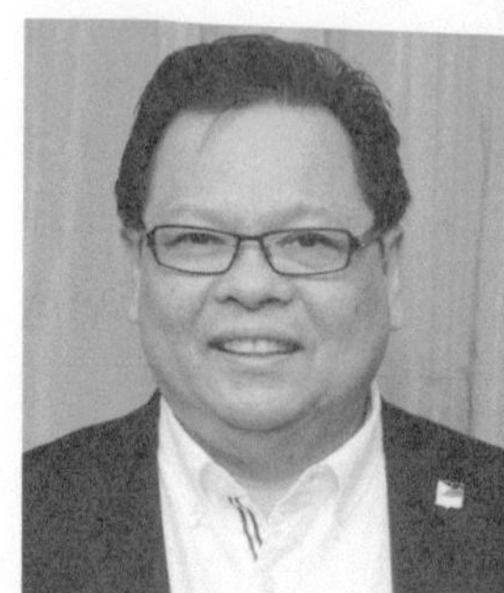
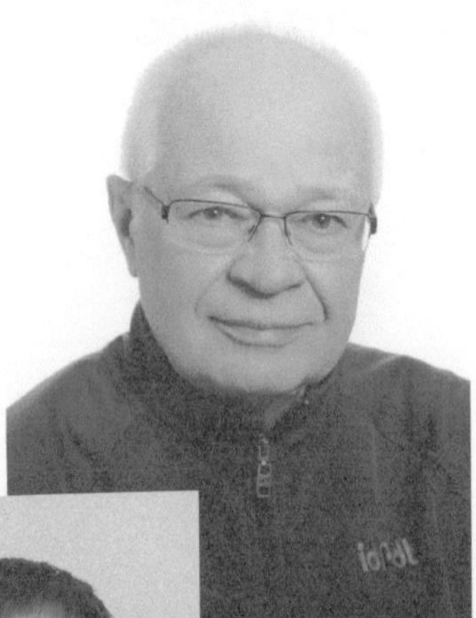
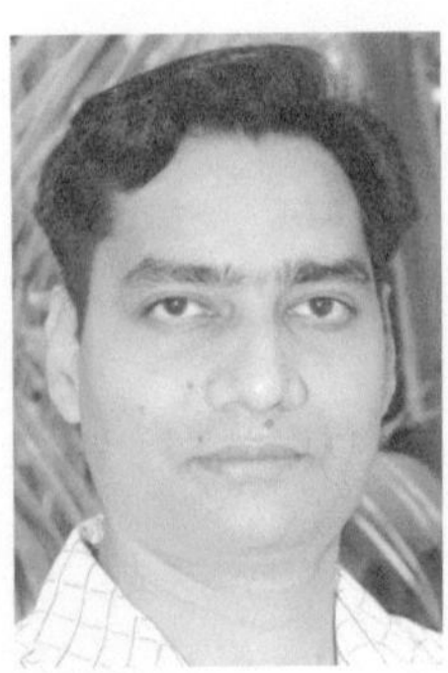
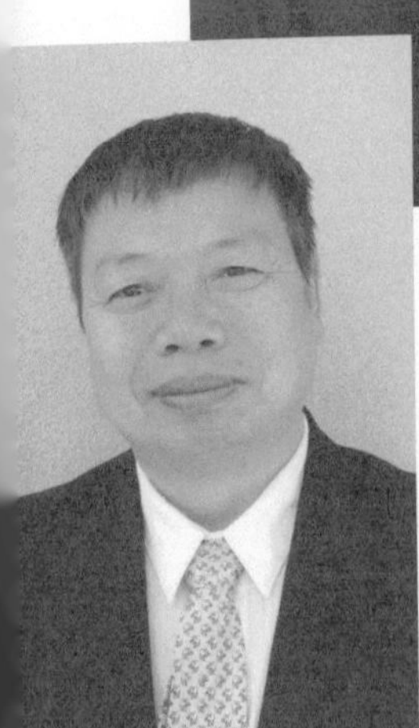
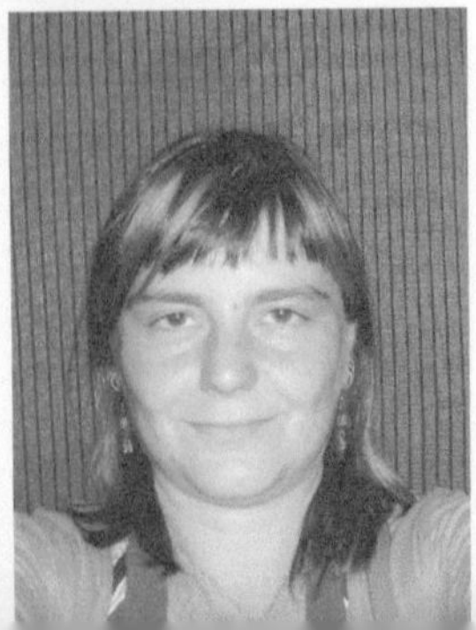
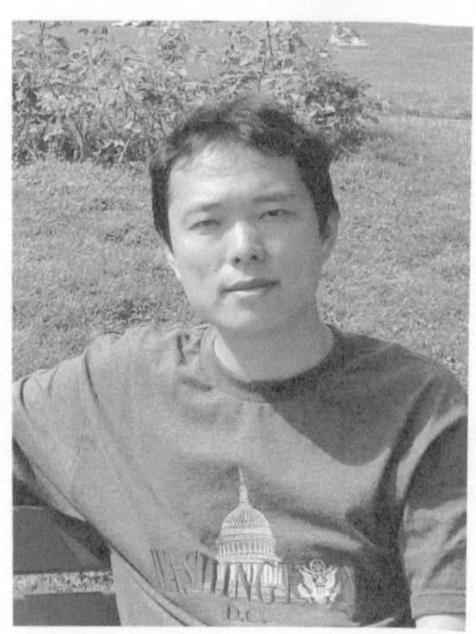

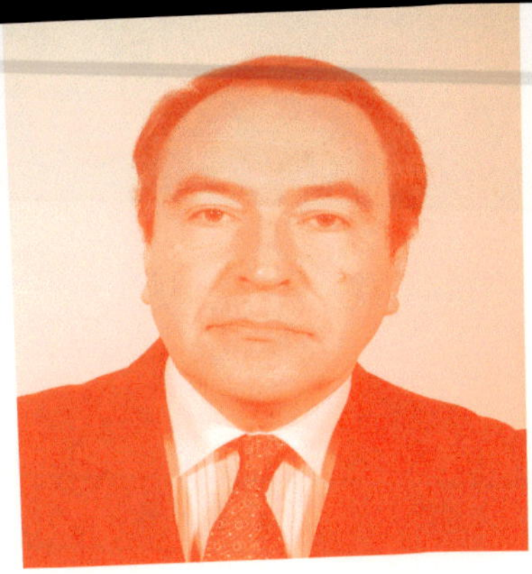
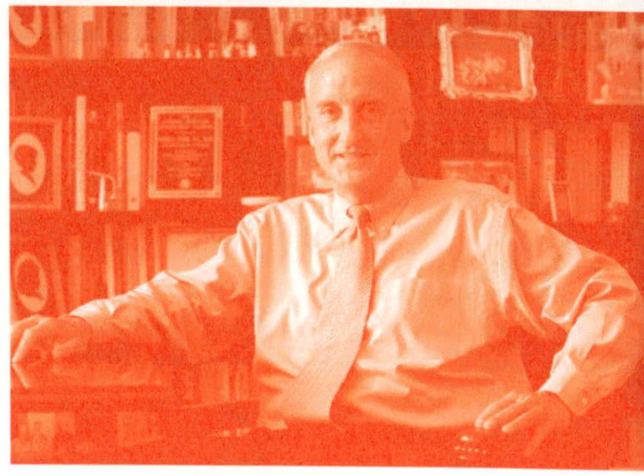
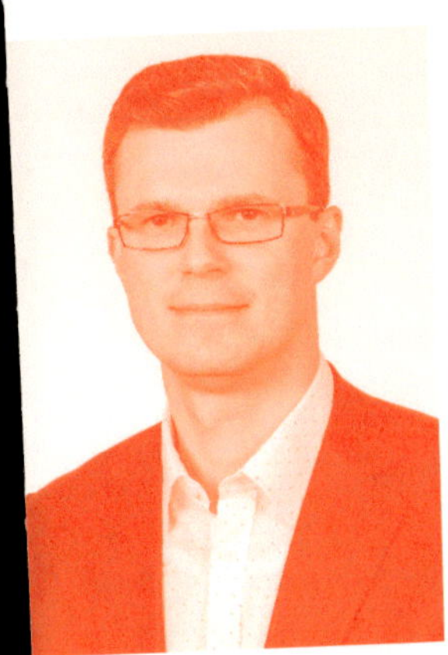
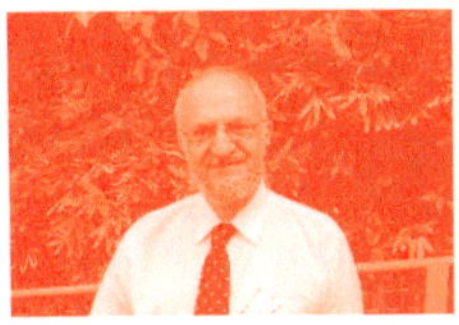
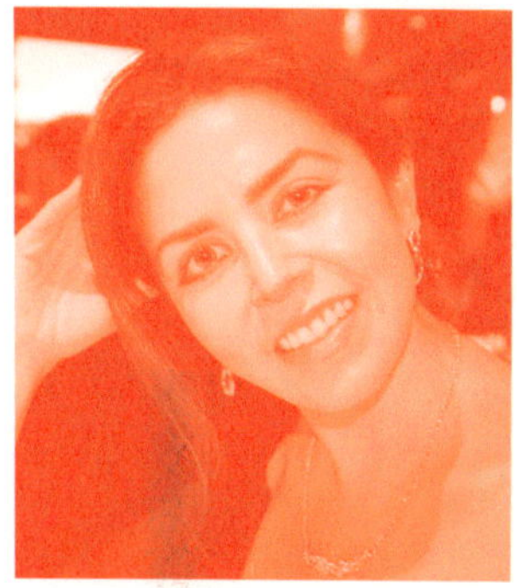

Supporting open minds since 2005

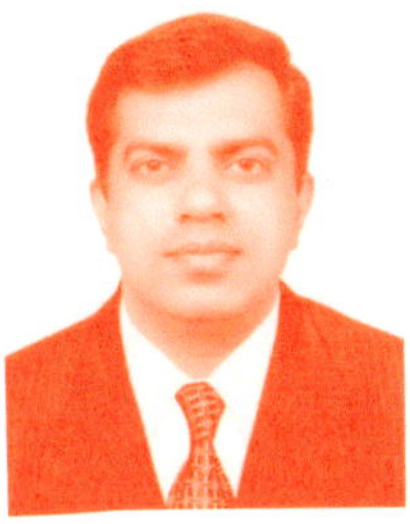
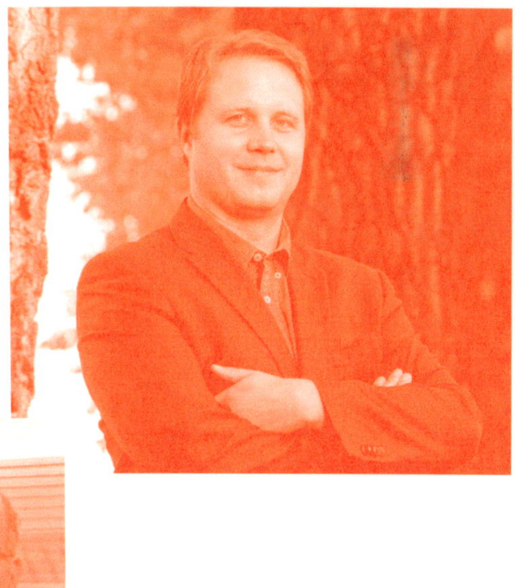
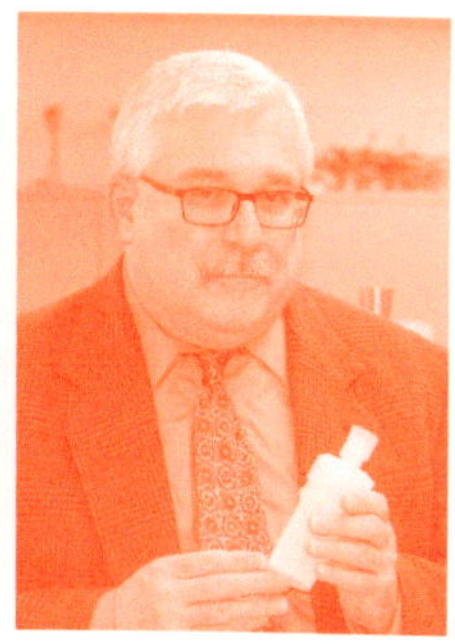
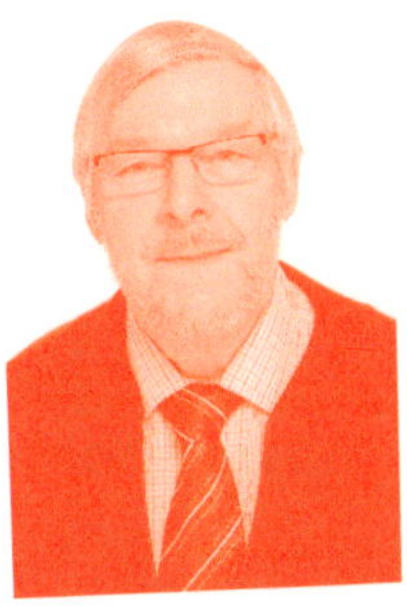
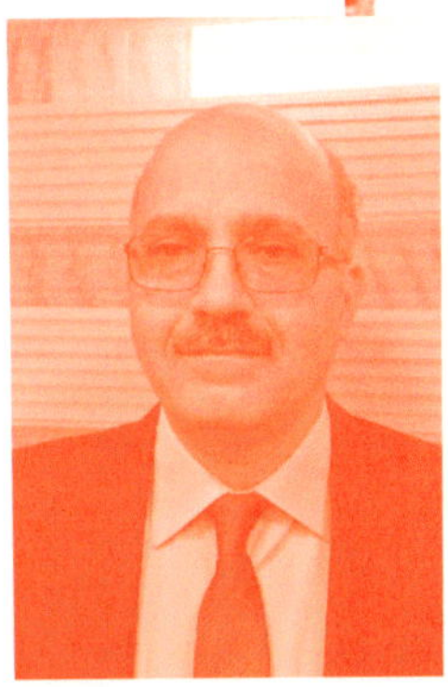
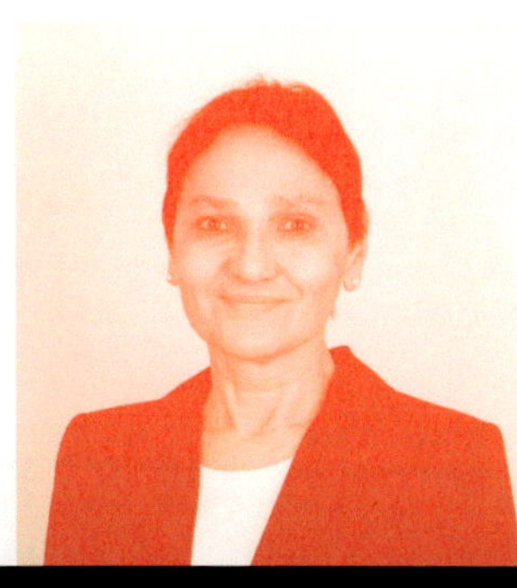
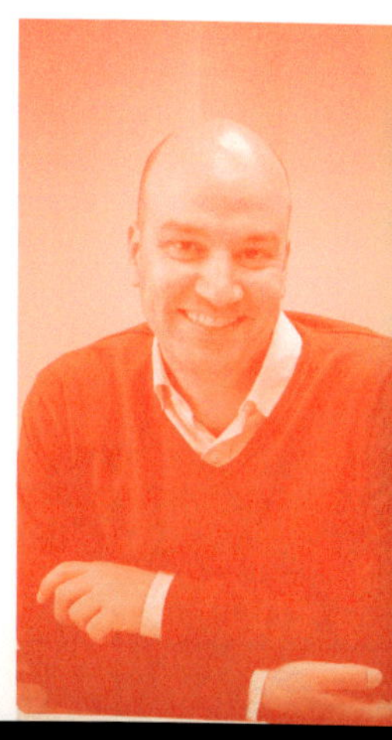

Artificial Intelligence in Oncology Drug Discovery and Development
http://dx.doi.org/10.5772/intechopen.88376
Edited by John W. Cassidy and Belle Taylor

Contributors
Dominic Magirr, Jacob Bradley, Roberta Dousa, Ayaka Shinozaki, John Cassidy, Kristofer Linton-Reid, Steve Gardner, Sayoni Das, Krystyna Taylor

First published in London, United Kingdom, 2020 by IntechOpen
IntechOpen is the global imprint of INTECHOPEN LIMITED, registered in England and Wales, registration number: 11086078, 7th floor, 10 Lower Thames Street, London, EC3R 6AF, United Kingdom
Printed in Croatia

British Library Cataloguing-in-Publication Data
A catalogue record for this book is available from the British Library

Additional hard and PDF copies can be obtained from orders@intechopen.com

Artificial Intelligence in Oncology Drug Discovery and Development
Edited by John W. Cassidy and Belle Taylor
p. cm.
Print ISBN 978-1-78984-689-8
Online ISBN 978-1-78985-897-6
eBook (PDF) ISBN 978-1-78985-898-3

An electronic version of this book is freely available, thanks to the support of libraries working with Knowledge Unlatched. KU is a collaborative initiative designed to make high quality books Open Access for the public good. More information about the initiative and links to the Open Access version can be found at www.knowledgeunlatched.org

For EU product safety concerns:
IN TECH d.o.o., Prolaz Marije Krucifikse Kozulić 3, 51000 Rijeka, Croatia, info@intechopen.com or visit our website at intechopen.com.

Meet the editors

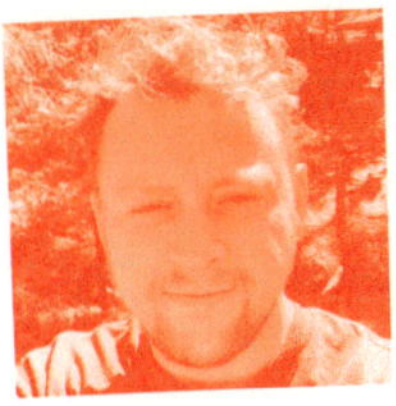

John Cassidy completed his PhD at the University of Cambridge, where his research focused on understanding and modelling the causes of tumour heterogeneity and how tumour evolution could impact clinical practice. In 2015, he founded CCG.ai to continue this mission and to apply advances in machine learning to the discovery of tumour biomarkers. In 2017, he was included on the prestigious Forbes 30 Under 30, and in 2020 was elected a fellow of the Royal Society of Biology. Dr. Cassidy sits on multiple advisory councils and boards both in the United Kingdom and internationally. He has published papers in journals such as *Cell and Cancer Research* and has helped raise more than £20m in grant funding for cancer research projects.

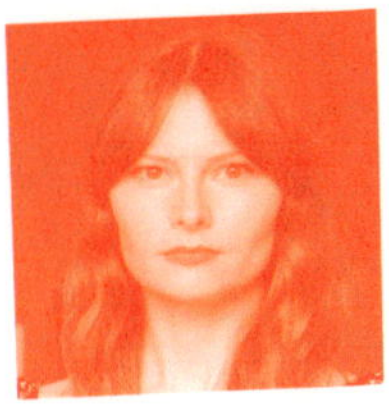

Belle Taylor is a communications and engagement professional, currently based at the University of Edinburgh. A chemist by training, she has a First Class Chemistry MSci from University College London (UCL), where she also undertook her PhD. As a science communicator, she regularly speaks at and chairs events across the country. She is also co-host of the science comedy show "Our Disgusting Planet."

Contents

Preface

Cancer remains one of the leading causes of morbidity and mortality worldwide. In 2020, we will have an estimated 15 million new diagnoses and 12 million new cancer-related deaths [1]. As we move further into the decades ahead, an increasing proportion of this global challenge will be shouldered by developing nations. This is part of a larger epidemiological shift as chronic, non-communicable disease—associated with diet, tobacco, alcohol, lack of exercise, and industrial exposures—is added to morbidities attributable to infectious disease in the world's emerging economies [2].

The cancer therapeutic market was estimated to reach $98.9 billion USD in 2018, with a compounded annual growth rate of 7.7%. The cost of individual cancer drugs is similarly rising at a rate well above inflation. Ipilimumab, for example, was priced at $120,000 on launch, despite providing an overall survival benefit of just four months. More generally, if we correct for inflation and increased survival benefit, the average cost of new cancer therapies increased $8,500 per year from 1995 to 2013 [3]. If we continue along this path of yearly incremental price increases in new therapies, whilst not seeing associated health benefits, public opinion may begin to further question the moral standing of the pharmaceuticals industry [4]. Moreover, will it really be sustainable to treat a worldwide increase in the incidence of cancer with more and more expensive drugs?

It is not simply a case of capping the price of essential medicines, or even seizing the means of production. Indeed, drug discovery and development are long and arduous processes; recent figures point to 10 years and $2 billion USD to take a new chemical agent from discovery through to market. Moreover, though an approved blockbuster drug can be lucrative for the controlling pharmaceutical company, new therapeutic agents suffer from a 90% attrition during development, making the chances of success in the drug development process low.

Nor is it as easy as developing better drugs. As our understanding of the importance of tumour heterogeneity and evolution continues to improve, it is becoming increasingly evident that new strategies may be needed to continue our fight against cancer [5, 6]. New therapeutic agents, such as immunotherapies, new strategies such as combination therapy and new ways of testing drugs such as adaptive clinical trials are all appropriate for tumour biology, but many orders of magnitude more expensive than standard chemotherapy.

Efficiency of drug discovery and development together with clinical testing and delivery of new medicines must improve by orders of magnitude if we are to keep pace with a growing understanding of tumour biology and a growing incidence of disease in the developing world. Thankfully, computational techniques such as machine learning (ML) and artificial intelligence (AI) have re-emerged in the last several years as powerful sets of tools for unlocking value from large datasets. ML has shown great promise in improving efficiencies across numerous industries with high-quality, vast, datasets. In an age of increasing access to highly curated rich sources of biological data, ML shows promise in reversing some of the negative trends shown in drug discovery and development. As biology in general and cancer research in particular become ever richer in data, there is a great deal of promise for ML in changing the cancer drug development landscape [7].

This book explores the role of AI and ML in improving the efficiency in drug discovery and development. In general, the contents should be accessible cross-disciplinarily to both cancer biologists and computer scientists, though we do zoom in to focus on some specific technical challenges, for example, in the structuring of genomic data (Chapter 3) and the interpretation of clinical trials (Chapter 6). As a particularly unique feature of this book, Chapter 8 deals with patients' perspectives on the free use of clinical data and the implementation of AI in the clinical workflow.

John W. Cassidy
Cambridge Cancer Genomics,
United Kingdom

Belle Taylor
University of Edinburgh,
United Kingdom

References

[1] Jemal A, Bray F, Center MM, Ferlay J, Ward E, Forman D. Global cancer statistics. CA: A Cancer Journal for Clinicians. 2011

[2] Kanavos P. The rising burden of cancer in the developing world. Annals of Oncology. 2006

[3] Howard DH, Bach PB, Berndt ER, Conti RM. Pricing in the market for anticancer drugs. Journal of Economic Perspectives. 2015

[4] Pollack A. Drug Goes From $13.50 a Tablet to $750, Overnight - The New York Times. The New York Times. 2015

[5] Cassidy JW, Batra AS, Greenwood W, Bruna A. Patient-derived tumour xenografts for breast cancer drug discovery. Endocrine-Related Cancer. 2016

[6] Cassidy JW, Caldas C, Bruna A. Maintaining tumor heterogeneity in patient-derived tumor xenografts. Cancer Research. 2015

[7] Cassidy JW. Studying the clonal origins of drug resistance in human breast cancers. University of Cambridge; 2019

Section 1

AI in Drug Development

Chapter 1

Introduction: An Overview of AI in Oncology Drug Discovery and Development

Kristofer Linton-Reid

Abstract

Artificial intelligence (AI) has been termed the machine for the fourth industrial revolution. One of the main challenges in drug discovery and development is the time and costs required to sustain the drug development pipeline. It is estimated to cost over 2.6 billion USD and take over a decade to develop cancer therapeutics. This is primarily due to the high numbers of candidate drugs failing at late drug development stages. Many sizable pharmaceutical and biotech companies have made considerable investments in AI. This is primarily due to recent advancements in AI, which have displayed the possibility of rapid low-cost drug discovery and development. This overview provides a general introduction to AI in drug discovery and development. This chapter will describe the conventional oncology drug discovery pipeline and its associated challenges. Fundamental AI concepts are also introduced, alongside historical and modern advancements within AI and drug discovery and development. Lastly, the future potential and challenges of AI in oncology are discussed.

Keywords: oncology, AI, drug discovery, drug development

1. Introduction

Artificial intelligence (AI) has been termed the machine for the fourth industrial revolution. AI is anticipated to transform every industry. In drug discovery and development, the key challenges are the time and costs required to sustain the drug development pipeline. It is estimated to cost over 2.6 billion USD and take over a decade to develop an oncology therapeutic [1]. These soaring costs are mostly a result of money invested in the 90% of candidate therapies that fail at the late stages of drug development, between phase 1 trials and regulatory approval [2]. AI is projected to be the foundation for an era of quicker, cheaper, and more efficient drug discovery and development.

Recent advancements in AI are displaying the possibility of rapid low-cost drug discovery and development. The term AI broadly describes the ability of a machine to perform tasks commonly associated with intelligent beings. Another term, machine learning (ML), is a subset of AI involving machines using data to artificially think for themselves. The main difference between ML and AI is that ML is the direct application and involves the combination and analysis of complex, disparate data sets.

Within the pharmaceutical industry, experts agree that AI will revolutionize and change how drugs are discovered. There are many components, directly and indirectly, related to the drug discovery and development that AI can enhance. These include but are not limited to: the use of AI in tumour classification [3], computer-aided organic synthesis [4], compound discovery [5], assay development, and biomarker and target discovery [6–8]. In general, AI aims to automate and optimize slow processes to substantially speed up the R&D drug discovery process.

Several pharmaceutical, biotech, and software companies are also making every effort to integrate AI with drug discovery and development. In 2016, Pfizer partnered with IBM Watson Health, an AI platform, to enhance their search for immuno-oncology treatments. Sanofi paired with Dundee university spin-out Exscientia, to discover metabolic-disease therapies. In 2009, Roche acquired Genentech for $46.8 billion, providing a foundation for Roche's biotechnology division, which is not integrating AI. Genentech is now collaborating with GNS Healthcare platform to use machine learning to find and validate potential new drug candidates. Recently, Genentech displayed the capacity of AI to diagnose diabetic macular degeneration.

Even large traditional tech companies are investing in drug development. Alphabet's subsidiary DeepMind developed an AI platform, AlphaFold, that predicted protein 3D structures based upon genomic data; their prediction was better than over 90 other companies including Novartis, and Pfizer, in the 13th Critical Assessment of Structure Prediction. DeepMind's success with AlphaFold is displaying how non-healthcare companies can also contribute to and improve the drug discovery and development pipeline. These investments are forming a clear vision that AI will play an important role in future drug discovery and development.

In this overview, we start with introducing key components of conventional oncology drug discovery, and associated shortfalls. Following this, fundamental AI concepts are introduced, alongside historical and modern advancements within AI and drug discovery and development. Lastly, the future potential and challenges of AI in oncology are introduced.

2. Conventional oncology drug discovery and development

The conventional drug discovery and development pipeline has five key components: target identification, lead discovery, preclinical development, clinical development, and regulatory approval (**Figure 1**). A drug discovery program initiates after researching the inhibition or activation of a protein or pathway and explaining the potential therapeutic effect. This leads to the selection of a biological target, often requiring extensive validation prior to the lead drug discovery phase. This phase involves the search for a viable drug-like small molecule or biological

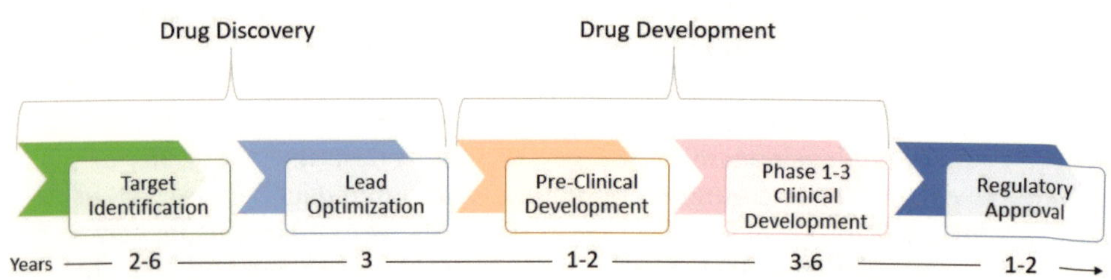

Figure 1.
Five key components of drug discovery and development: target identification, lead discovery, preclinical development, clinical development, and regulatory approval.

therapy, termed a development candidate. The drug candidate will progress into preclinical development, and if successful into clinical development.

2.1 Drug discovery and development pipeline: target identification and validation

Biological target identification and validation is a fundamental step in drug discovery. A biological target is a broad term, used to describe a variety of entities including proteins, metabolites, and genes. A biological target must have a clear effect, meet clinical and therapeutic needs, as well as industry needs. Above all, a biological target must be 'druggable'. The term 'druggable' refers to a target that can be bound by a small molecule or larger biologic and elicit a response.

2.1.1 Target identification

A variety of methods exist to identify biological targets. This includes gene expression, proteomics and genomics analysis, and phenotypic screening.

The analysis of mRNA/protein expression is often employed to elucidate expression to disease relationships if changes in expression levels are correlated with exacerbation or progression. At the genetic level, targets are identified by determining if there is an association between genetic polymorphism and disease occurrence or progression. For example, one of the most well-studied genetic-disease associations is that of *N*-acetyltransferase 2 (*NAT2*) with bladder and colon cancer. *N*-acetyltransferase 1 (*NAT1*) and *NAT2* are precursors of enzymes that mediate the transformation of two types of carcinogens, aromatic and heterocyclic amines. The *NAT2* rapid acetylator phenotype and the slowest NAT2 acetylator phenotype are associated with colon and bladder cancer respectively [9, 10].

Phenotypic screening is another method for target identification. This can take a variety of forms. Generally, compounds are screened in cellular or animal disease models to identify a compound that leads to the desired change in phenotype. Kurosawa and colleagues [11] screened for overexpressed carcinoma antigens by isolating human monoclonal antibodies that bind to the surface of tumour cells. In this study, clones were screened with immunostaining. Clones that displayed strong staining with the malignant cells were selected. Subsequently, 21 distinct antigens were derived via mass spectroscopy. Several immunotherapies may be capable of binding to these 21 antigen targets, possibly leading to a new clinical therapy.

Target identification may involve one or a combination of the previously mentioned methods.

2.1.2 Target validation

While identifying a target typically requires one method, the following target validation requires a variety of methods. A multi-validation approach increases confidence in the biological target and subsequent drug candidate's success.

There are a variety of target validation methods that may be implemented, although validation almost always requires target expression in the disease-relevant cells or tissues. A typical primary validation protocol is to measure the expression of protein and/or mRNA in clinical samples, with immunohistochemistry and in situ hybridization.

Generally, in vivo studies are often a pivotal factor in the decision to proceed with drug development; these usually involve protein inhibition/gene knock-out/knock-in studies. Transgenic animal models are particularly useful as they facilitate phenotypic observations. These animal models often yield insights into potential therapeutic side effects. Transgenic models traditionally gene edits whereby an animal would lack or obtain a certain gene(s) for its entire life. An example is the P2X7 knockout mouse model, which lacks an inflammatory and neuropathic response. These knockout mice revealed their respective mechanism of action, as their cells did not release the mature pro-inflammatory cytokine IL-1beta from cells, despite IL-1 beta expression remaining constant. Contrary to gene knockout models, are gene knock-ins models. In gene knock-ins, genes not originally in the mouse are inserted, and subsequent disease protein is synthesized. These transgenic animals usually have a different phenotype to a knockout and may mimic more closely what happens during disease and treatment.

Another in vivo technique used for target identification is antisense oligonucleotide-based models. Antisense oligonucleotides mimic RNA and complement the target mRNA molecule [12]. Bound antisense oligonucleotide prevents ribosomal translation of mRNA to protein. Honore and colleagues created an antisense oligonucleotide that inhibited translation of the rat P2X3 receptor [13]. When rat models were dosed with P2X3 antisense, they displayed anti-hyperalgesic activity. Once administration of the antisense oligonucleonucleotides was discontinued, receptor function and algesic responses returned. Unlike transgenic model, the antisense oligonucleotide effect is reversible [14].

While there are many viable target validation methods, two modern technologies can enable tissue specific validation: clustered regularly interspaced short palindromic repeats (CRISPR), and CRISPR-related techniques, and organs on a chip.

The CRISPR-Cas9 and related approaches provide multiple advancements compared to the transgenic model; these include the ability to overcome embryonic lethality and avoid resistance mechanisms. In brief, CRISPR-Cas9 works by distributing the Cas9 nuclease into the cell. Synthetic guide RNA then guides the nuclease to the desired cut location, facilitating the addition or removal of genes in vivo [15]. An example of CRISPR-Cas 9 target validation is with the elucidation of the mechanism of action behind tumour suppressor, p53, reactivating compounds. Employing CRISPR-Cas9-based target validation in lung and colorectal cancer displayed that the anti-proliferate activity of nutlin is dependent on functional p53. However, using traditional models, the mechanism and therapeutic response to p53-reactivating compounds is lost via compound-specific resistance mechanisms [16].

Another emerging technology that will facilitate improved target validation is organs-on-chips. These are multi-channel 3-D microfluidic cell culture chips that mimic the functionality and physiology of entire organs. This technology yields the potential to quickly assess the efficacy and human response to target mediation. Song and colleagues used a vasculature system chip model to assess the relationship between vascular endothelium and the metastatic behavior of circulating tumour cells. This study suggested that the inhibition of CXCL12-CXCR4 binding on endothelial cells may be a valid target in the prevention of metastasis [17]. Importantly, organs-on-chips technologies may provide novel insights to target identification and validation studies.

Overall, there are many means to validate targets; all strategies have a common aim: to evaluate the target's cellular function prior to full investment into the target, and drug candidate screening.

2.2 Drug discovery and development pipeline: lead discovery

Once the biological targets have been identified and validated, the next fundamental step is the lead discovery phase. This comprises of three components, in order: hit identification, hit-to-lead phase, and lead optimization.

2.2.1 Drug discovery and development pipeline: hit identification

It is during this phase that drug compound screening assays are developed, and subsequent 'hit' compounds derived. The term 'hit' compound is used in a range of terminologies; in this overview we refer to it as a compound that obtains the desired screening effect, which has been validated upon retesting. Various screening approaches exist to identify hit molecules. In this overview, we will describe the most common screening strategies: high throughput screening, Focused based screening, and fragment screening.

High throughput screening utilizes an entire compound library and assesses the activity of each compound on the biological target. This typically involves large semi-automated cell-based assays. A candidate hit compound typically requires further assays to confirm its mechanism of action [18].

Focused based screening, also termed knowledge-based screening, selects compounds from a library based on existing information about the target, stemming from literature or patents, which suggest compounds likely to yield the desired target activity [19].

Fragment screening uses small-molecular weight compound libraries and screens these compounds at high concentrations. Small fragments that bind to the target are often scaled with chemical alterations to increase their binding affinity [20].

2.2.2 Hit-to-lead phase and lead optimization

The aim of this intermediate phase is to develop a compound(s) with enhanced properties, with pharmacokinetics suitable for one or many different in vivo models. This step regularly involves a series of structure-active-relationship (SAR) investigations for each hit compound, in an attempt to measure the activity and selectivity of each compound.

The goal of the final lead discovery phase is to obtain compounds with optimal structural, metabolic, and pharmacokinetic properties. This often involves further applications of various in vitro and in vivo screens.

2.3 Drug discovery and development pipeline: preclinical

Once a lead candidate is identified, further elucidation of its structure, metabolic, and pharmacokinetic properties may be required. The typical preclinical development stage is comprised of various components, typically used with animal models: (1) The first preclinical experiments revolve around dose design; a safe dose must be identified with estimated human measurements. (2) Second, the pharmacodynamics of a compound is required; the mechanism of action that causes the clinical response, with respect to doses, must be determined. (3) Third, pharmacokinetics properties of the drug candidate are required. This includes absorption, distribution, metabolism, excretion, and potential drug-drug interactions. The aim of preclinical studies is to obtain enough information to determine a safe dose for the first human study. On average, one in 5000 preclinical development candidate drugs make it through preclinical development and become regulatory approved [21].

2.4 Drug discovery and development pipeline: clinical development

The clinical development/clinical trial stage comprised of three main stages and one post-market surveillance stage.

The phase 1 clinical studies are carried out in a small number of healthy volunteers. The aim of this stage is to distinguish a therapy's metabolic and pharmacological effects, as well as the side effect response to varying dosages. The main aim of phase 1 is to determine a therapy's safety profile.

Stemming from the data collected during phase 1, phase 2 studies also termed 'therapeutic exploratory' trials involve investigations on several diseased individuals. This phase aims to further determine the effectiveness of the drug with respect to disease or condition. Side effects and risks are further distinguished. Phase 2 studies are controlled, usually conducted on a few hundred patients.

The phase 3 studies are a much larger drug assessment of the drug's efficacy, safety, and evaluate the overall benefit-risk relationship of the drug. This phase may also yield enough data to estimate the results of a general population, as they include several hundred to several thousand people.

Once the drug is approved, there is a fourth phase, known as post-marketing surveillance. These are observational studies, whereby the goal is to define and ensure the safety profile of the drug on a larger population scale.

2.5 Drug discovery and development pipeline: challenges and overview

There are three main reasons why drugs fail: the first is that they simply do not work, second is that they are unsafe for clinical use, and the third reason of drug failure is due to poor clinical trial structure. The cost of a candidate soars the further it gets in the drug development pipeline.

The primary source of trial failure is a drug's lack of efficacy. Hwang and colleagues investigated 640 phase 3 trials, of which 54% failed. Over 50% of these failures were due to a lack of efficacy [22]. There are a variety of reasons why a drug may enter phase 3 trials and yet lack efficacy. This may also include the propagation of error due to flawed target validation, a poor study design, or simply having an insufficient number of patient trials resulting in weak statistical power and an inability to reject the null hypothesis.

The infamous, poly ADP ribose polymerase (PARP) inhibitor, Olaparib failed its first trial for ovarian cancer due to a lack of trial structure. In the initial trial, in individuals with the BRCA mutation and platinum-sensitive recurrent ovarian cancer, Olaparib delayed the time to recurrence to 11.2 months from 4.3 months. However, the median time to death was 34.9 months in the treatment group and 31.9 months in the control group ($p = 0.19$) [23]. In 2014, Olaparib was approved by the FDA for women with recurrent ovarian cancer who have the germline *BRCA* mutation and had previously received three or more lines of chemotherapy. This approval was based on a study by Kaufman and colleagues [24], which displayed a response rate > 30% with Olaparib monotherapy in patients who had previously received three or more lines of chemotherapy.

Clinical trials also fail with respect to safety. In Hwang and colleagues' study, out of the initial 640 compounds, 17% of them failed due to safety [22]. Drug safety is a key factor in every stage of the candidate drug development; however, challenges may only present at larger populations [25]. One reason for failure due to safety is due to ill reporting of safety concerns. Generally, a patient's safety concerns may not align with that of the administering physician. It is logical to assume people will be more likely to report an adverse event that is of concern to them. It is important that at each step within the drug development pipeline safety is a primary consideration. The cost of determining a safety issue propagates with progression through each drug development stage.

One of the most impactful drug candidate failures was with sulphanilamide. This drug was popular in the 1930s and sold in both a bolus and elixir form. However, important safety tests had not been conducted for the elixir form,

DOI: http://dx.doi.org/10.5772/intechopen.92799

although at the time this testing was not required. Unfortunately, after being treated with the elixir form, over 100 people died due to diethylene glycol poisoning [26]. This led to the implementation of two important acts: The Food, Drug and Cosmetic Act and Drugs and Cosmetics Act.

3. The potential of AI

AI has been utilized in drug discovery since the early 1960s. However, in 2016 many large pharmaceutical companies started investing in AI by partnering with AI startups or academic groups or initiating their own internal AI R&D programs. This has resulted in an enormous number of new publications within the field that cover the entire drug discovery and development pipeline. This has included the implementation of deep learning models to predict the properties of small molecules from transcriptomics data [27] to the identification of novel drug targets [28]. AI has integrated into almost every area of drug discovery and development.

The primary aim of drug discovery and development combined with AI remains to facilitate the development of the best drugs and bring them to the clinic to fulfill unmet medical needs.

AI and machine learning has a lot of potential. For those new to the field, AI limitations seem endless, regardless of the input information. AI has a range of applications. It can be successful at creating an image of a cat from a model trained on images of cats or can enable a car to drive automatically without making a single mistake, or a drug that can be designed to treat a disease safely and efficaciously. However, AI will not succeed with every challenge; it is simply a tool that may drive new technologies, and enhanced understanding. In drug discovery and development, AI is not one entity that can design a drug from start to finish, but many different AIs which enhance our understanding throughout the drug discovery and development process.

3.1 Fundamental AI concepts

While many computational approaches can fit the broad definition of AI, two fields are currently popular: machine learning and its subfield deep learning. In layman's terms, the key difference with deep learning is that it uses multiple layers, each employing different calculations on the initial data. In order to understand their capacities, a few fundamental concepts must be understood.

Broadly, there are two different types of machine learning to understand. Supervised learning is when a model is trained using labeled data sets to predict a certain outcome. An example of this is the quantitative structure–activity relationship (QSAR) approach. This is used to predict a chemical's property, such as solubility and bioactivity [29]. The other approach is unsupervised learning, as the name suggests, it does not depend upon training with labeled data to find relationships with data. Examples include the use of hierarchical clustering, algorithms and principal components analysis to analyze and group large molecular libraries into smaller sub-groups of similar compounds.

With supervised machine learning, there are two types: classification and regression. Classification models are used when the problem is categorical, as in the predicted output is a limited set of values. Regression models are used when the problem involves predicting a numeric value within a range.

There are a variety of different types of machine learning models, such as random forests, autoencoders, and convolutional neural networks. Each of the subsequent chapters will describe specific models as required.

3.2 Examples of AI implementations in drug discovery and development

A vast number of AI and drug discovery papers are published every day, covering various aspects of the entire drug discovery and development pipeline. Drug discovery and development-based AI technologies range from the identification and validation of drug targets, drug repurposing, identification of new compounds, and improving the R&D efficiency. There are a number of potential contributions AI can make to reduce inefficiencies in the conventional drug development and discovery pipeline.

Target identification and validation have been enhanced by AI. This is made possible by genomics, with biochemical and histopathological information. The IBM Watson identified five novel RNA-binding proteins as potential targets linked to the pathogenesis of amyotrophic lateral sclerosis, which currently has no known cure [30].

One huge opportunity for AI in drug discovery is with drug repurposing. As an example, Donner and colleagues [31] used a transcriptomics data set and derived a new measurement of compound functionality, based on gene expression. This measurement allowed the identification of compounds that shared biological targets, despite being structurally different, revealing previously unknown functional associations between compounds.

An AI platform that can predict a candidate's mechanism of action and in vivo safety would cut wasted costs dramatically. There are several examples of companies with this goal. This includes DeeoTox and ProCTOR, both of which aim to predict the toxicity of new compounds [32, 33]. The performance of these AI platforms is expected to increase as larger robust data sets on the toxicity of compounds are made available.

As of 2019, one important study was the discovery of a drug within 21 days. Deep learning enabled the identification of potent DDR1 kinase inhibitors within 21 days. Out of the four compounds discovered, one lead candidate has displayed ideal pharmacokinetics in mice [34].

Overall, it is clear AI may yield increases in drug discovery efficiency through various strategies.

3.3 Current challenges in AI

AI has shown promise in drug discovery and development. However, it is not without its challenges. There are many challenges faced by AI in medical research such as lack of data, lack of interoperability, and the curse of dimensionality.

The lack of data is a recurring problem throughout every industry wanting to implement AI. The minimum number of samples in a traditional biological study is five, for it to be valid. However, most machine learning algorithms must be trained on hundreds, or thousands, of data points/samples, in order to perform well. Furthermore, obtaining labeled data can be a challenge, as this often requires some form of manual input. Fortunately, large databases, such as The Cancer Genome Atlas program (TCGA), are aggregating and open-sourcing vast amounts of robust data from multiple institutions. However, on some occasions, large databases that include the requested data may not exist. One such strategy to combat this is data augmentation. Data augmentation is the process of creating artificial data from real data. There are a variety of data augmentation approaches; ultimately they increase the data available for training models, without collecting new data.

Another challenge faced by machine learning is the lack of interpretability. The term 'black box model' is often used when it is difficult to explain how a model makes certain predictions and performs. This is more likely an occurrence with deep learning, as each layer adds complexity to the model explaining each layer's outputs

DOI: http://dx.doi.org/10.5772/intechopen.92799

can become exponentially complex and the number of layers increases. However, a variety of tools are being developed in order to elucidate further explainability such as LIME (Local Interpretable Model-Agnostic Explanations) and SHAP (Shapley Additive Explanations). LIME adopts a local linear approximation of the model's behavior, whereas SHAP employs a game theory-based approach to explain the model output. Both LIME and SHAP, and other similar strategies, are projected to become common practice in machine learning and are going to be necessary to get more AI technologies to the clinic [35].

A recurring issue with artificial intelligence in medical data is known as the curse of dimensionality. This is when the data sets used have a small number of samples and many features. This is a common occurrence in medical omics data sets, as they typically yield thousands of features and less than 100 samples; thus the available data become sparse. This problem may be addressed with a variety of dimensionality reduction techniques.

Overall, there are a series of challenges that will need to be addressed for AI to reach its optimal capacity. In this passage, we have only described a few challenges. However, they are being addressed with advancements in complementary data science approaches and tools, such as the creation of large data repositories, tools to increase explainability, and the creation of feature reduction techniques.

4. Concluding remarks

Taking a drug from idea to the clinic is a long diverse process, costing over 2.6 billion dollars, and take over a decade to develop a cancer therapeutic. This is primarily due to high numbers of candidate drugs failing at late drug development stages. Advancements in AI are continually displaying the possibility of rapid low-cost drug discovery and development. As we make our way through the 2020s, it is evident the drug discovery and development will be permanently shaped by AI.

Acknowledgements

The author would like to thank N.B.N and I.H.

Conflict of interest

The author declares no conflict of interest.

Acronyms and abbreviations

AI	artificial intelligence
CRISPR	clustered regularly interspaced short palindromic repeats
ML	machine learning
NAT1	*N*-acetyltransferase 1
NAT2	*N*-acetyltransferase 2
PARP	poly ADP ribose polymerase
TCGA	The Cancer Genome Atlas

Author details

Kristofer Linton-Reid
Imperial College London, London, UK

*Address all correspondence to: kl2418@ic.ac.uk

References

[1] Avorn J. The $2.6 billion pill—Methodologic and policy considerations. New England Journal of Medicine. 2015;**372**:1877-1879. DOI: 10.1056/NEJMp1500848

[2] Seyhan AA. Lost in translation: The valley of death across preclinical and clinical divide—Identification of problems and overcoming obstacles. Translational Medicine Communications. 2019;**4**:1-19. DOI: 10.1186/s41231-019-0050-7

[3] Tripathy RK, Mahanta S, Paul S. Artificial intelligence-based classification of breast cancer using cellular images. RSC Advances. 2014;**4**:9349-9355. DOI: 10.1039/c3ra47489e

[4] Zhou Z, Li X, Zare RN. Optimizing chemical reactions with deep reinforcement learning. ACS Central Science. 2017;**3**:1337-1344. DOI: 10.1021/acscentsci.7b00492

[5] Popova M, Isayev O, Tropsha A. Deep reinforcement learning for de novo drug design. Science Advances. 2018;**4**:eaap7885. DOI: 10.1126/sciadv.aap7885

[6] Hofmarcher M, Rumetshofer E, Clevert DA, Hochreiter S, Klambauer G. Accurate prediction of biological assays with high-throughput microscopy images and convolutional networks. Journal of Chemical Information and Modeling. 2019;**59**:1163-1171. DOI: 10.1021/acs.jcim.8b00670

[7] Klambauer G, Hochreiter S, Rarey M. Machine learning in drug discovery. Journal of Chemical Information and Modeling. 2019;**59**:945-946. DOI: 10.1021/acs.jcim.9b00136

[8] Yin Z, Ai H, Zhang L, Ren G, Wang Y, Zhao Q, et al. Predicting the cytotoxicity of chemicals using ensemble learning methods and molecular fingerprints. Journal of Applied Toxicology. 2019;**39**:1366-1377. DOI: 10.1002/jat.3785

[9] Hein DW. Molecular genetics and function of NAT1 and NAT2: Role in aromatic amine metabolism and carcinogenesis. Mutation Research. 2002;**506-507**:65-77. DOI: 10.1016/s0027-5107(02)00153-7

[10] Golka K, Prior V, Blaszkewicz M, Bolt HM. The enhanced bladder cancer susceptibility of NAT2 slow acetylators towards aromatic amines: A review considering ethnic differences. Toxicology Letters. 2002;**128**:229-241. DOI: 10.1016/s0378-4274(01)00544-6

[11] Kurosawa G, Akahori Y, Morita M, Sumitomo M, Sato N, Muramatsu C, et al. Comprehensive screening for antigens overexpressed on carcinomas via isolation of human mAbs that may be therapeutic. Proceedings of the National Academy of Sciences of the United States of America. 2008;**105**:7287-7292. DOI: 10.1073/pnas.0712202105

[12] Taylor MF, Wiederholt K, Sverdrup F. Antisense oligonucleotides: A systematic high-throughput approach to target validation and gene function determination. Drug Discovery Today. 1999;**4**:562-567. DOI: 10.1016/S1359-6446(99)01392-6

[13] Honore P, Kage K, Mikusa J, Watt AT, Johnston JF, Wyatt JR, et al. Analgesic profile of intrathecal P2X3 antisense oligonucleotide treatment in chronic inflammatory and neuropathic pain states in rats. Pain. 2002;**99**:11-19. DOI: 10.1016/S0304-3959(02)00032-5

[14] Miller CM, Harris EN. Antisense oligonucleotides: Treatment strategies and cellular internalization. RNA & Disease. 2016;**3**(4):e1393. DOI: 10.14800/rd.1393

[15] Hendel A, Bak RO, Clark JT, Kennedy AB, Ryan DE, Roy S, et al. Chemically modified guide RNAs enhance CRISPR-Cas genome editing in human primary cells. Nature Biotechnology. 2015;**33**:985-989. DOI: 10.1038/nbt.3290

[16] Wanzel M, Vischedyk JB, Gittler MP, Gremke N, Seiz JR, Hefter M, et al. CRISPR-Cas9-based target validation for p53-reactivating model compounds. Nature Chemical Biology. 2016;**12**:22-28. DOI: 10.1038/nchembio.1965

[17] Song JW, Cavnar SP, Walker AC, Luker KE, Gupta M, Tung Y-C, et al. Microfluidic endothelium for studying the intravascular adhesion of metastatic breast cancer cells. PLoS ONE. 2009;**4**:e5756. DOI: 10.1371/journal.pone.0005756

[18] Entzeroth M, Flotow H, Condron P. Overview of high-throughput screening. Current Protocols in Pharmacology. 2009. Chapter 9: Unit 9.4. DOI: 10.1002/0471141755.ph0904s44

[19] Boppana K, Dubey PK, Jagarlapudi SARP, Vadivelan S, Rambabu G. Knowledge based identification of MAO-B selective inhibitors using pharmacophore and structure based virtual screening models. European Journal of Medicinal Chemistry. 2009;**44**:3584-3590. DOI: 10.1016/j.ejmech.2009.02.031

[20] Price AJ, Howard S, Cons BD. Fragment-based drug discovery and its application to challenging drug targets. Essays in Biochemistry. 2017;**61**:475-484. DOI: 10.1042/EBC20170029

[21] Umscheid CA, Margolis DJ, Grossman CE. Key concepts of clinical trials: A narrative review. Postgraduate Medicine. 2011;**123**:194-204. DOI: 10.3810/pgm.2011.09.2475

[22] Hwang TJ, Carpenter D, Lauffenburger JC, Wang B, Franklin JM, Kesselheim AS. Failure of investigational drugs in late-stage clinical development and publication of trial results. JAMA Internal Medicine. 2016;**176**:1826-1833. DOI: 10.1001/jamainternmed.2016.6008

[23] Ledermann J, Harter P, Gourley C, Friedlander M, Vergote I, Rustin G, et al. Olaparib maintenance therapy in patients with platinum-sensitive relapsed serous ovarian cancer: A preplanned retrospective analysis of outcomes by BRCA status in a randomised phase 2 trial. The Lancet Oncology. 2014;**15**:852-861. DOI: 10.1016/S1470-2045(14)70228-1

[24] Kaufman B, Shapira-Frommer R, Schmutzler RK, Audeh MW, Friedlander M, Balmaña J, et al. Olaparib monotherapy in patients with advanced cancer and a germline BRCA1/2 mutation. Journal of Clinical Oncology. 2015;**33**:244-250. DOI: 10.1200/JCO.2014.56.2728

[25] Crowther M. Phase 4 research: What happens when the rubber meets the road? Hematology/The Education Program of the American Society of Hematology American Society of Hematology Education Program. 2013;**2013**:15-18. DOI: 10.1182/asheducation-2013.1.15

[26] Paine MF. Therapeutic disasters that hastened safety testing of new drugs. Clinical Pharmacology and Therapeutics. 2017;**101**:430-434. DOI: 10.1002/cpt.613

[27] Aliper A, Plis S, Artemov A, Ulloa A, Mamoshina P, Zhavoronkov A. Deep learning applications for predicting pharmacological properties of drugs and drug repurposing using transcriptomic data. Molecular Pharmaceutics. 2016;**13**:2524-2530. DOI: 10.1021/acs.molpharmaceut.6b00248

[28] Li Q, Lai L. Prediction of potential drug targets based on simple sequence properties. BMC

Bioinformatics. 2007;**8**:1-11. DOI: 10.1186/1471-2105-8-353

[29] Cherkasov A, Muratov EN, Fourches D, Varnek A, Baskin II, Cronin M, et al. QSAR modeling: Where have you been? Where are you going to? Journal of Medicinal Chemistry. 2014;**57**:4977-5010. DOI: 10.1021/jm4004285

[30] Bakkar N, Kovalik T, Lorenzini I, Spangler S, Lacoste A, Sponaugle K, et al. Artificial intelligence in neurodegenerative disease research: Use of IBM Watson to identify additional RNA-binding proteins altered in amyotrophic lateral sclerosis. Acta Neuropathologica. 2018;**135**:227-247. DOI: 10.1007/s00401-017-1785-8

[31] Donner Y, Kazmierczak S, Fortney K. Drug repurposing using deep Embeddings of gene expression profiles. Molecular Pharmaceutics. 2018;**15**:4314-4325. DOI: 10.1021/acs.molpharmaceut.8b00284

[32] Gayvert KM, Madhukar NS, Elemento O. A data-driven approach to predicting successes and failures of clinical trials. Cell Chemical Biology. 2016;**23**:1294-1301. DOI: 10.1016/j.chembiol.2016.07.023

[33] Mayr A, Klambauer G, Unterthiner T, Hochreiter S. DeepTox: Toxicity prediction using deep learning. Frontiers in Environmental Science. 2016;**3**:80. DOI: 10.3389/fenvs.2015.00080

[34] Zhavoronkov A, Ivanenkov YA, Aliper A, Veselov MS, Aladinskiy VA, Aladinskaya AV, et al. Deep learning enables rapid identification of potent DDR1 kinase inhibitors. Nature Biotechnology. 2019;**37**:1038-1040. DOI: 10.1038/s41587-019-0224-x

[35] Ribeiro MT, Singh S, Guestrin C. "Why should i trust you?" Explaining the predictions of any classifier. In: Proceedings of the ACM SIGKDD International Conference on Knowledge Discovery and Data Mining, vol. 13-17, August-2016, Association for Computing Machinery. 2016. pp. 1135-1144. DOI: 10.1145/2939672.2939778

Chapter 2

Applications of Machine Learning in Drug Discovery I: Target Discovery and Small Molecule Drug Design

John W. Cassidy

Abstract

Drug discovery and development are long and arduous processes; recent figures point to 10 years and $2 billion USD to take a new chemical agent from discovery through to market. Moreover, though an approved blockbuster drug can be lucrative for the controlling pharmaceutical company, new therapeutic agents suffer from a 90% attrition during development, making the chances of success in the drug development process relatively low. Machine learning (ML) has re-emerged in the last several years as a powerful set of tools for unlocking value from large datasets. ML has shown great promise in improving efficiencies across numerous industries with high quality, vast, datasets. In an age of increasing access to highly curated rich sources of biological data, ML shows promise in reversing some of the negative trends shown in drug discovery and development. In this first part of our analysis of the application of ML to the drug discovery and development process, we discuss recent advances in the use of computational techniques in drug target discovery and lead molecule optimisation. We focus our analysis on oncology, though make reference to the wider field of human health and disease.

Keywords: cancer, machine learning, drug discovery, computational biology

1. Introduction

Cancer is, first and foremost, a disease of the genome. Specific changes in the DNA of an otherwise normal cell, caused by environmental mutagens or as a result of a defective DNA repair mechanisms, result in inherited base-pair changes in the genome of daughter cells [1]. Such mutations can be benign (i.e. 'passenger mutations') or can directly contribute to malignant transformation of the cell (i.e. 'driver mutations') [2, 3]. Over the past few decades, advances in our understanding of these basic principles have led to unprecedented clarity in the genomic drivers of tumour development. Projects such as The Cancer Genome Atlas [4] and International Cancer Genome Consortium [5] have sequenced thousands of cancers and systematically classified common mutations into driver or passenger categories. Concurrently, advances in our understanding of the context of these mutations, for example through the advent of high throughput methylome sequencing [6] and the numerous studies on the functional consequences of a mutation for cell signalling [1], have helped us design therapeutic strategies to halt tumour progression.

Specifically, whereas some of the earliest cancer drugs were serendipitously discovered and functioned through the inhibition of cell division on an organism-wide scale, increasingly, new molecular agents are designed to specifically inhibit the function of single molecular targets driving tumour growth [7]. The first of these molecularly targeted drugs for cancer were developed in the 1970s and 1980s. These 'targeted therapies' have many notable success stories, such as Gleevec (for BCR-ABL positive leukaemia), Herceptin (for *Erbb2* amplified breast cancer) and Tamoxifen (for ER positive breast cancer) [1, 8–10]. As we enter the 2020s, the oncology pharmaceutical industry is now producing >60 new molecularly targeted cancer therapies per year.

Although each of these targeted therapies has the potential to generate billions of dollars in revenue for their parent pharmaceutical company, typically there is a 90% attrition rate between Phase I clinical trials and market approval; additionally, each drug may cost $2.6 billion USD to go from target identification to approval [11, 12]. Interestingly, the difference between a so-called blockbuster drug (one generating >$1 billion a year in gross revenues) and a market failure, is arguably almost entirely based on patient cohort selection. An interesting case study comes from Olaparib, the first in a class of *poly ADP ribose polymerase* (PARP) inhibitors developed by KuDOS Therapeutics after initial work from the Stephen Jackson, amongst others, and ultimately taken through clinical trials by AstraZeneca. Olaparib activates a 'synthetic lethality' pathway in *Brca1/2* mutant breast cancers by biasing DNA-damaged cells toward double strand breaks rather than mismatch repair pathways [13]. *Brca1/2* mutations are common in triple negative breast cancer (TNBC) and the initial clinical trials sought to leverage the efficacy of Olaparib in *Brca1/2* mutant TNBCs to show increased overall survival in all TNBCs. These initial trials failed, primarily because patient stratification was sub-optimal. The use of ML in improving patient stratification through the identification of complex biomarkers of clinical response will be discussed in depth in the latter part of this series: *Applications of Machine Learning in Drug Discovery II: Biomarker Discovery, Patient Stratification and Pharmacoeconomics*.

Like the above Olaparib example, and the preceding examples of success in targeted therapy more generally, the pre-emanant strategy in drug discovery is first to establish a causal relationship between a gene, mutation, or pathway and pathophysiological features of a disease [14]. Although other strategies, such as phenotypic screening [12], have witnessed a resurgence in popularity recently, this rational target discovery is still heavily relied upon in drug discovery programs the world over. Typically, once a target has been identified and its causal role in disease progression confirmed through, for example gene perturbation studies, a molecule is sought to perturb the targets function (or abnormal function) whilst having minimal effect on other proteins [15]. These molecules can be rationally designed if the three-dimensional structure of the target protein is known, we can screen a large library of small molecules with drug-like properties, or we can use a technique such as phage display to identify monoclonal antibody species with specific inhibitory function.

Complicating matters somewhat, perturbation of a molecular target can be inhibitory (i.e. antagonist), excitatory (i.e. agonist), excitatory of a secondary downstream pathway (i.e. biased agonist) or be inhibitory of the basal effects of target activity (i.e. inverse agonist). Moreover, small molecules may bind to protein clefts with known activity or function (e.g. an ATP-binding pocket) or secondary allosteric sites of unknown function in the protein or even its surroundings.

There are therefore at least three stages in early drug development which could be advanced by computational approaches such as ML: (1) target identification from literature data mining, (2) structure-based design of drugs intended to perturb a target, and (3) optimisation of screening protocols for small molecule or biologic inhibitors. In this chapter, we will provide a basic primer to ML before discussing methods for, and examples of, the use of ML-based techniques in target identification and structure-based drug design.

2. Machine learning—a primer

Fundamentally, ML is the design and deployment of statistical models used to parse large datasets, learn from underlying patterns present in the data and apply those learnings to make predictions about future data [16]. This differs fundamentally from many rule-based algorithms in that the predictive power of the model is improved when exposed to more data, rather than necessarily when any expert understanding is improved. The strength of ML is to solve problems for which large, well annotated, datasets exist but for where the underlying connection between variables in the dataset is unknown. For these reasons, the application of ML to the field of modern biology is extremely well suited.

A core objective of any ML model is to generalise from experience, *i.e.* to accurately predict some aspect of an unseen dataset after training on a prior dataset. Before selecting a model to use in a particular situation, we must have methods for determining its performance. To assess our model, we must be cognisant of the required parameter tuning and the overall separation of signal from noise [16]. As we cannot sample all possible futures, and because training sets are, by definition, finite, we typically must express performance in terms of probabilistic bounds. Numerous probabilistic evaluation metrics are commonly used by the field for drawing comparisons between models, for example classification accuracy, kappa, area under the curve (AUC), logarithmic loss and confusion matrix the F1 score [14, 17, 18]. Additionally, the available of gold standard datasets are invaluable for testing new model performance.

In optimising for model performance, we must also be cognisant of overfitting to the data, which occurs when a model attempts to include and account for dataset noise in the hypothesis, which can significantly impact model generalisation. Formally, the complexity of a model's hypothesis should match that of the function underlying the dataset. Underfitting occurs when the hypothesis is less complex that the underlying function, and overfitting occurs when the hypothesis is too complex.

In practice, there are a number of technical methods for dealing with overfitting. For example, we can hold back part of the training dataset to use as a validation dataset. This process can be automated and randomised for each new model build, so long as each model is trained on one subset of the data and tested on another, unseen, subset. We can also account for fit in our model design, for example by adding 'penalties' to model performance for each new parameter is incorporated into the model. This process is known as regularisation and forces models to generalise without overfitting to the data, examples in practice include Ridge, LASSO and elastic nets [16, 19, 20].

Of course, there are many different models which we can train on a single dataset, we can avoid brute force sensitivity and specificity optimisation by understanding some of the philosophy underlying different model architectures. Broadly, we can define ML models as being either supervised or unsupervised, named for the datasets for which the methods work. In supervised learning, the model is a mathematical relationship between variables found in a dataset with known input and output variables (for example drug treatment and patient outcome) [15, 21]. We then ask the model to predict future outputs for unseen inputs.

The most well-known example of supervised learning is a linear regression between two known variables; however, models can be significantly more complicated. Unsupervised learning, on the other hand, finds patterns hidden within input data and builds clusters based on intrinsic structures or relationships between data points. Of course, there is a great deal of nuance between supervised (with completely labelled training data) and unsupervised (without any labelled training data). Indeed, combining the two model types on the same dataset (semi-supervised learning) is increasingly employed in the field [21].

ML models themselves are numerous and varied; and our goal here is not to present a comprehensive library of models. However, because of their increasing popularity in the field, artificial neural networks (ANNs) deserve special mention. ANNs belong to their own subset of ML methods known as Deep Learning [22–24]. Deep Learning models are inspired by biological neural networks in that they are comprised of many connected nodes ('neurons'), with each connection transmitting 'signal' between nodes, like a synapse. Typically, this signal is a number, and each neuron performs some non-linear function of the sum of its inputs. As the network completes several attempts at 'learning' a task, the mathematical weighting of each nodal connection is determined based on that node's contribution to a successful outcome [24]. In this way, the ANN is thought to resemble the function of biological synapse restructuring during a learning task. Unlike a biological brain, neurons in the ANN are arranged in layers, with each layer performing a specific task or data transformation. ANNs and Deep Learning in general have been successful in a variety of tasks, from computer vision and mobile advertising to cancer variant detection and patient outcome prediction [17, 23, 25].

3. ML for target identification

Aside from purely phenotypic screening approaches, the typical target discovery process begins with target identification and prioritisation. As discussed, this requires identification of a target with a causal link with some aspect of a pathophysiology and a plausible framework for believing that modulation of this target will result in modulation of the disease itself [14, 15]. Though proof of a successful therapeutic strategy will come first from *in vivo* drug response studies and ultimately through showing efficacy in a randomised clinical trial, there is no doubt that target identification is a crucial step in this path.

The first full DNA genome to be sequenced was that of a bacteriophage, completed in 1977 [26]. This catalysed a multinational effort to sequence the human genome, which was completed by 2001 at a cost of >$1 billion [27]. Around this same time, commercial sequencers had begun to become available and what has become known as Next Generation Sequencing (NGS) began to be carried out in labs across the world. What has followed is the age of big biological data. As the price of sequencing continues to fall, we have seen projects such as The Cancer Genome Atlas [4] that publish thousands of genomes. Recently, this has been extended to national scale projects such as the UK's 100,000 Genome Project [28] and the beginning of an age of incorporating genomics into the regular clinical workflow for cancer patients, pioneered by the likes of Memorial Sloan Kettering with their *Integrated Mutation Profiling of Actionable Cancer Targets* (IMPACT) study [29]. Alongside this surge in genomics, we have seen unprecedented development of other high-throughput technologies in cancer research, from RNA-sequencing to methylome sequencing and imaging-based proteomics [1].

Cumulatively, these efforts have transformed biology from a functional low-throughput pursuit to one which is increasingly rich in data. The ability to mine these datasets in target discovery efforts has been democratised through an increasing willingness amongst researchers to share data. However, finding meaningful patterns in such multi-dimensional data requires statistical models of sufficient complexity to yield meaningful results. Such tasks are perfectly suited for ML-based techniques.

Perhaps the richest untapped resource in new therapeutic target discovery is the scientific literature itself, representing countless years of experimental data from groups around the world. However, these largely unstructured data present several challenges. Recent advances in the field of natural language processing (NLP) have gone some way to resolving these issues. For example, Kim and colleagues developed an NLP-based tool for disease-gene relationship building from unstructured Medline abstracts [30]. Biological events between genes and disease types are extracted and these associations are ranked based on the strength of evidence sentences using a Bayesian classifier. This tool, named DigSee, identified associations between 13,054 genes and 4494 disease types, which the authors claim is more than any manually curated database currently available. Although difficult to verify the associations, the authors further showed that these relationships were at least comparable to those inferred from such manually curated databases [30].

ML can also be useful in the prediction of unseen biology. For example, Costa and colleagues built a computational model to predict morbid genes (i.e. those where mutations could cause hereditary human disease) and druggable genes (i.e. those coding for proteins able to be modulated by small molecules to elicit a phenotypic effect) on a genome wide scale [31]. Such efforts have the potential to reduce laborious experimental procedures and identify early likelihood of a putative molecular target to be causally associated with disease. The authors trained a decision tree-based meta-classifier on databases of protein–protein, metabolic and transcriptional interactions, as well as tissue expression and subcellular localization for known morbid or druggable genes. Although the meta-classifier had questionable results, correctly recovering just 65% of known morbid genes (precision 66%) and 78% of known druggable genes (precision 75%), the authors were able to inspect the decision tree and uncover rules for morbidity and druggability [31]. Parameters such as membrane localisation (for druggability) and regulation by multiple transcription factors (for morbidity), suggesting that the model was correctly identifying biological traits.

A more common approach is to focus on a specific disease or therapeutic area. For example, Jeon and colleagues built a support vector machine (SVM) classifier that integrated a variety of genomic and systematic datasets to classify proteins based on their likelihood to bind a small molecule drug and prioritised targets specific for breast, pancreatic and ovarian cancer [32]. Like Costa et al., the classifier developed appears to have uncovered biological rational from a data-driven perspective; Key classification features were gene essentiality, mRNA expression, DNA copy number, mutation occurrence and protein-protein interaction network topology [31, 32]. The authors then designed therapeutic strategies and validated their targets using proliferation-based assays in cancer cell line models with either synthetic peptides or small molecule inhibitors. In total, the authors found 122 putative tumour-type-agnostic targets, 69 of which overlapped with known cancer targets, together with 266 specific to breast, 462 to pancreatic and 355 to ovarian cancer [32].

Although many diseases are known to be monogenic, many more are associated with dysregulation of complicated multi-genomic signalling pathways [11]. Designing a therapeutic strategy in this case can be aided by taking a systems biology approach. Ament and colleagues followed such rational when they reconstructed a transcription factor regulatory network associated with pre-symptomatic

Huntington's disease [33]. This genome scale model carried information on the target genes of a total of 718 distinct transcription factors associated with mouse models of the disease. The authors selected a regression model with LASSO regularisation to avoid overfit and discovered a total of 48 differentially expressed TF-target gene modules associated with age- and CAG repeat length-dependent gene expression changes in *Htt* CAG knock-in mouse striatum [20, 34]. Of these, 13 were further validated in human samples and the authors experimentally validated one based on the transcription factor SMAD3.

Taking the concept of target identification in complicated disease states further, Mamoshina and colleagues took advantage of advances in the discovery of biomarkers of in muscle tissues to find druggable targets underpinning the molecular basis of human ageing [35]. The authors constructed an SVM-based model with linear kernel and deep feature selection to identify gene expression signatures associated with ageing. The model's performance was evaluated on gene expression samples from the Gene expression Genotype-Tissue Expression (GTEx) project and achieved an accuracy of 0.80 when predicting the binned age, highlighting the importance of external gold-standard datasets in model tuning [36]. Importantly, the model confirmed several established mechanisms of human skeletal muscle ageing, including neurotransmitter recycling, IGFR and PI3K-Akt-mTOR signalling and dysregulation of cytosolic Ca^{2+} homeostasis, giving a biological basis for the model's effectiveness [35]. Moreover, the model generated a set of targets with druggable properties, suggesting future therapeutic intervention may be possible.

4. ML for optimisation of high throughput screens

Once a target with causal relation to a disease phenotype of interest has been identified, the next step is typically to identify and optimise a suitable chemical entity to perturb the normal or pathogenic activity of said target. Until very recently, by far the most common approach to identify such candidate molecules was through a high throughput screen (HTS). Typically, a suitable reporter system would be designed, exposed to a pharmaceutical company's vast compound libraries and any reporter changes reported. For example, in the task of identifying antagonists for the β2 adrenoceptor, researchers may design a radioligand binding assay whereby a library of new chemical agents are assayed for their ability to interfere with radiolabelled fenoterol (an agonist) and radiolabelled alprenolol (an antagonist) binding. Characteristics of their binding (e.g. K_D as a measure of affinity) correspond to changes in surface plasmon resonance (SPR) detected at the receptor [37], allowing researchers to select a variety of candidate molecules into the lead optimisation phase.

An alternative use of HTS techniques, which is becoming ever more important, is phenotypic screening. Here, researchers look for a specific phenotypic change induced by one of the thousands of screened chemicals against a process or cell type of interest. In the most simplistic sense, we could be screening for cell death in a heterogenous cell population [12], but more complicated indicators (such as fluorescence activated by signalling pathways) are in use in drug discovery processes across the industry [38]. As our understanding of tumour biology grows, researchers are increasingly favouring drug screens which preserve some degree of tumour heterogeneity, thus complicated phenotypic screens are growing in importance in drug discovery [1].

Advanced imaging is a popular technique for identification of complex phenotypes and perturbations, and can be greatly enhanced by the use of advanced ML-based analytics. Broadly, we can think of imaging-based screens as composing of two camps. In the first, typically called high-content or phenotypic screening, we focus on pre-defined phenotypes and the candidate drugs which modulate it. For example, identification of compounds which modulate the subcellular localisation of specific pre-defined intracellular signalling molecules with a role in disease [39].

Alternatively, we may stain multiple subcellular structures with multiplexed fluorescent dyes or antibodies and expose cells to genetic, pathogenic or chemical perturbing agents and categorise their response. Such investigatory screens are highly amenable to automated image acquisition and analysis through machine learning. In order to profile phenotypes of cells in an unbiased manner, computer vision can be used to extract multivariant feature vectors of cellular morphology (size, shape, texture) as well as staining intensity. After cellular segmentation, feature sets of cells or groups of cells can then be stratified to find relationships between thousands of different perturbations which can give insights into mechanisms or action of drugs or help researchers piece together pathway information [40, 41].

In one study, Perlman and colleagues made multidimensional measurements of individual cell states for a variety of perturbations. The authors were able to build a multidimensional classifier to group small molecules with similar mechanism of action [42]. This technique has similarly been applied to correlate phenotypic response with chemical structure similarity by Young and colleagues [43]. In this study, researchers explored 'factor analysis' for large data reduction whilst retaining relevant biological information, then clustered their identified features into seven phenotypic categories containing compounds of similar mechanism of action and chemical structures. These techniques can be built upon to build annotated libraries of pharmacologically active small molecules and model their potential off-target affects *in silico* [44].

Moreover, the use of mechanisms of action association studies in high content imaging and HTS opens up drug repurposing and new target identification. For example, Breinig and colleagues used high-content screening and image analysis to measure effects of >1200 pharmacologically active compounds on complex phenotypes in isogenic cancer cell lines which had been genetically modified in key oncogenic signalling pathways [41]. The cell lines were exposed to a library of ~200 known drugs and phenotypic response recorded by high content imaging. The resource was published as the Pharmacogenetic Phenome Compendium (PGPC), to enable researchers to explore drug mechanisms of action, detect potential off-target effects, and generate hypotheses on drug combinations. The resource was validated by confirming that tyrphostin (EGFR inhibitor) has off-target activity on the proteasome [41].

5. ML for structure-based drug design

As discussed previously, after suitable target identification, a new therapeutic program relies on the discovery and development of one, or several, lead molecules which can perturb the targets normal structure [14]. Though traditionally these lead compounds were invariably small molecules, modern biology and particularly modern oncology relies on novel drug modalities. To modulate the function of a receptor molecule such as the adrenoreceptor (a G-protein coupled receptor) we require a molecule which resembles the structure of the natural ligand (in this case noradrenalin), but with some small functional changes [45]. However, many appealing drug targets have no such ligand binding domain (for example PARP), may activate in the absence of ligand [e.g. *the epidermal growth factor receptor* (EGFR)], may have no known ligand (e.g. HER2) or may bind many natural ligands (e.g. CXCR2) and thus any small molecule inhibitor could have cross-reactivity with other receptors [9, 13, 46–49]. These limitations have led to a multitude of drug targeting strategies, broadly described as 'biologics'. In cancer these include, humanised monoclonal antibodies, chimeric receptors, bi-specific antibodies, oncolytic viruses, and even engineered T-Cells, to name but a few [9, 38, 50–52]. Notwithstanding these advances, there are still a multitude of small molecule drugs developed each year.

Structure-based drug design (SBDD) typically begins with resolution of the three-dimensional structure of the target protein [53]. Traditionally, this process was the exclusive domain of experimental structural biology, through labour intensive tools such as nuclear magnetic resonance (NMR), X-ray crystallography, and cryo-electron microscopy [54]. However, modern computational techniques have opened up the possibility of *in silico* protein structure modelling [22]. Amongst such techniques, homology modelling, which begins with the known structure of a protein with >40% homology to the target, is often seen as the most reliable. Validation of a homology modelled structure is typically carried out by considering stereochemical properties in, for example, a Ramachandran plot [22]. Next, potential binding sites are modelled by considering interaction energy across the length of the folded protein when exposed to charged functional groups. Stable conformations are predicted with, for example, Q-SiteFinder, an energy-based method for binding site prediction [55]. Amino acid residues associated with putative binding sites can then be annotated for function.

Extensive virtual and experimental high-throughput screens (HTS) are then carried out against the synthesised or computationally modelled target protein with large compound libraries of drug like structures [53]. Candidates, or 'hits', in SBDD have stable free energies on docking with binding clefts on the target protein [56]. Alternatively, *de novo* drug design may be employed if the binding pocket is of sufficient resolution [57]. Hits then have their structures optimised against a set of ideal pharmacodynamic, pharmacokinetic and toxicological criteria. These processes are highly amenable to augmentation by ML based techniques.

For example, many studies have attempted to implement ANNs to ligand-based virtual screens, to varying levels of success. One such implementation of a multitask deep ANN was released by Ramsundar and colleagues as an open source tool known as DeepChem [58]. In general, multitask models outperform standard ANNs by synthesising information from many distinct sources. DeepChem itself powers ligand screening for commercial drug discovery with a simple python scripts to construct, fit, and evaluate sophisticated models [58]. The authors aimed to overcome barriers associated with software accessibility amongst the drug discovery industry. Moreover, their validation results demonstrated that multitask ANNs were robust and showed substantial improvements over more traditional techniques such as random forests. To help in benchmarking, a large library of 700,000 compounds and their binding data was collated by Wu and colleagues, and integrated into DeepChem [59].

When combining multitask ANNs, Markov state models and one-shot learning to reduce the data requirement of making meaningful predictions in a new experimental setup, we can identify previously unknown mechanisms of ligand receptor interaction [60]. For example, Farimani and colleagues performed extensive molecular dynamic simulation and analysis to find selective allosteric binding sites for the μ-opioid receptor, an important G-protein coupled receptor (GPCR) in analgesia [61]. Discovering novel allosteric sites is particularly relevant in analgesia and GPCR biology as new therapeutic agents could allow receptor modulation or fine-tuning without competing for receptor occupancy of the natural ligand.

ANNs can also be used to predict pharmacokinetic drug properties. In a competition sponsored by Merck, Sharp & Dohme, ANNs outperformed random forests and other ML methods in 13 of 15 assay-based classification tasks to predict absorption, distribution, metabolism and excretion (ADME) parameters of drug like molecules [62]. A multitask ANN also won the Tox21 dataset challenge of computational toxicity prediction of 12,000 compounds in 12 high-throughput toxicity assays. This ANN, developed by Mayer et al., and named DeepTox, normalises chemical structures computes chemical descriptors to train an ANN to predict the nuclear toxicity [63].

In addition to virtual screening and optimisation of lead compounds, we can use ML-based techniques to enhance *de novo* drug design by generating completely novel chemical entities. For example, Kadurin and colleagues combined variational autoencoders with generalised adversarial networks (GANs) to computer design highly selective and novel anticancer agents [64]. GANs are particularly interesting in *de novo* drug design; they function by training two ANNs (the generator and the discriminator) simultaneously with different and opposing objective functions. The GAN must compete in a zero-sum game to create a single best molecular structure [64]. A key preceding step is to use variational autoencoders to map chemical structures from known databases in latent space, the latent vector then transforms the molecular structure into a simplified molecular-input line-entry system (SMILES) string.

6. ML for drug repurposing

As discussed previously, the development of new drugs is a long and arduous process, often costing >$2 billion and taking 10 years. Even in phase III trials, drugs can fail because of some unforeseen side effect or off target affect. Interestingly, this very property opens up a shortcut for drug development. Over the last several years there has been substantial interest in repurposing existing drugs for new indications. This can be hypothesis driven, where we learn new features of a diseases pathology which make us confident that an existing inhibitor could be useful, or data driven, where researchers and companies use structure activity relationships to find serendipitous matches between known disease targets and already approved (or close to approval) drugs.

Various approaches underpinned by ML have been used to predict potential repurposing positions for drugs. For example, multiple studies have used natural language processing to make sense of text mined from electronic health records, clinical trial data and drug side-effect labels [15]. Correlation between drug molecules and clinicopathological symptoms, expression profiles or target pathway modulation can then be uncovered using a variety of ML techniques. In one study, for example, Zhao and So built drug-specific expression maps from transcriptomic changes collected from three cell lines exposed to a variety of compounds [65]. This method is powerful as the underlying mechanism of action of the drug need not be known. The authors could then apply a variety of ML models including deep neural networks, SVMs, elastic nets and gradient boosted machines to identify repositioning opportunities. However, the authors relied on cancer cell lines in this study, despite focussing on neurological conditions, we should be careful when extrapolating studies with inappropriate model systems [11].

Many academic and commercial groups have turned to a technique known as signature reversion (also known as connectivity mapping) in repurposing studies. Here, gene expression measurements by proteomics or transcriptomics are taken for various pathological phenotypes and built into, for example, graph networks of genewise expression changes. The objective is then to identify drugs which revert the genewise expression networks toward baseline. Driven by the desire to increase the drug development process for all concerned, researchers have been forthcoming in submitting such maps to open large-scale perturbation databases, such as Connectivity Map (CMap) or Library of Integrated Network-based Cellular Signatures (LINCS). Such databases have provided significant opportunities for computational pharmacogenomics and drug design [66].

It is worth noting that the majority of drug repurposing studies rely on an assumption that drugs with a similar chemical structure will behave in a similar fashion. This misconception has led to significant societal detriment in the past, for example in the thalidomide disaster. Thalidomide exists as two chiral forms (same chemical composition but having mirrored structures), one can be used to treat morning sickness; the other has teratogen effects.

7. Conclusion

ML is a powerful technique for identifying hidden patterns in complex datasets. Although based on standard statistical methods, recent advances in available compute power have led to a resurgence of the field. Deep Learning, in particular, has seen a profound resurgence in popularity and has the potential to revolutionise multiple fields of human endeavour. As we increasingly move into an age of large medical datasets, from clinical studies to massive cell line -omics databases, there is clearly an opportunity for application of machine learning to biology. Amongst biological problems, there is a pressing need for increased efficiency of the drug discovery process, particularly in high mortality and morbidity problems like oncology. For these reasons, we have seen significant steps toward the application of ML to cancer drug discovery over the past several years. In this chapter, we have discussed some of these efforts, including the use of ML for target identification and in structure-based drug design. Additionally, we have provided a primer to ML in an effort to familiarise biologists to the field. In the second part of our work, addressed in the second part of our analysis (*Applications of Machine Learning in Drug Discovery II: Biomarker Discovery and Patient Stratification*), we extend the analysis of uses of ML in the drug discovery process to the clinical arena. First, we will discuss the use of ML in biomarker discovery, before moving to clinical trial optimisation and post market treatment effectiveness monitoring.

Author details

John W. Cassidy
University of Cambridge, The Old Schools, Trinity Lane, Cambridge, CB21TN, UK

*Address all correspondence to: john.cassidy1@me.com; john@ccg.ai

References

[1] Cassidy JW. Studying The Clonal Origins of Drug Resistance in Human Breast Cancers. Cambridge University Press; 2019

[2] Akbar A, Dubourg-Felonneau G, Solovyev A, Cassidy JW, Patel N, Clifford HW. Effective sub-clonal cancer representation to predict tumor evolution. Mach Learn Heal [Internet]. 28 November 2019;**2**(1):12-17. Available from: http://arxiv.org/abs/1911.12774 [cited: 23 February 2020]

[3] Bozic I, Antal T, Ohtsuki H, Carter H, Kim D, Chen S, et al. Accumulation of driver and passenger mutations during tumor progression. Proceedings of the National Academy of Sciences of the United States of America. 2010;**107**(43):18545-18550

[4] Weinstein JN, Collisson EA, Mills GB, KRM S, Ozenberger BA, Ellrott K, et al. The cancer genome atlas pan-cancer analysis project. Nature Genetics. 2013;**45**:1113-1120

[5] Berger D. International cancer genome consortium. Im Focus Onkologie. 2013;**16**(5):49

[6] Koboldt DC, Fulton RS, McLellan MD, Schmidt H, Kalicki-Veizer J, McMichael JF, et al. Comprehensive molecular portraits of human breast tumours. Nature. 2012;**32**(12):324-432

[7] Cassidy JW, Bruna A. Tumor heterogeneity. In: Patient Derived Tumor Xenograft Models: Promise, Potential and Practice. Academic Press; 2017. pp. 37-55

[8] Capdeville R, Buchdunger E, Zimmermann J, Matter A. Glivec (ST1571, imatinib), a rationally developed, targeted anticancer drug. Nature Reviews Drug Discovery. 2002;**1**:493-502

[9] Nahta R, Esteva FJ. Herceptin: Mechanisms of action and resistance. Cancer Letters. 2006;**232**:123-138

[10] Abe O, Abe R, Enomoto K, Kikuchi K, Koyama H, Masuda H, et al. Relevance of breast cancer hormone receptors and other factors to the efficacy of adjuvant tamoxifen: Patient-level meta-analysis of randomised trials. Lancet. 2011;**34**(3):345-465

[11] Cassidy JW, Caldas C, Bruna A. Maintaining tumor heterogeneity in patient-derived tumor xenografts. Cancer Research. 2015:132

[12] Bruna A, Rueda OM, Greenwood W, Batra AS, Callari M, Batra RN, et al. A biobank of breast cancer explants with preserved intra-tumor heterogeneity to screen anticancer compounds. Cell. 2016;**167**(1):260-274.e22

[13] Lord CJ, Ashworth A. PARP inhibitors: Synthetic lethality in the clinic. Science. 2017;**355**:1152-1158

[14] Lavecchia A. Machine-learning approaches in drug discovery: Methods and applications. Drug Discovery Today. 2015:356-366

[15] Vamathevan J, Clark D, Czodrowski P, Dunham I, Ferran E, Lee G, et al. Applications of machine learning in drug discovery and development. Nature Reviews Drug Discovery. 2019:367

[16] Tiwari AK. Introduction to machine learning. Ubiquitous Machine Learning and Its Applications. 2017. pp. 1-14

[17] Dubourg-Felonneau G, Cannings T, Cotter F, Thompson H, Patel N, Cassidy JW, et al. A framework for implementing machine learning on omics data. Mach Learn Heal [Internet]. 26 November 2018;**1**(1):3-10. Available from: http://arxiv.org/abs/1811.10455 [cited: 23 February 2020]

[18] Dubourg-Felonneau G, Kussad Y, Kirkham D, Cassidy JW, Patel N, Clifford HW. Learning embeddings from cancer mutation sets for classification tasks. Mach Learn Heal [Internet]. 20 November 2019;**3**(1):1-12. Available from: http://arxiv.org/abs/1911.09008 [cited: 23 February 2020]

[19] Zou H, Hastie T. Regularization and variable selection via the elastic net. Journal of the Royal Statistical Society: Series B (Statistical Methodology). 2005;**67**(2):301-320

[20] Tibshirani R. Regression shrinkage and selection via the lasso. Journal of the Royal Statistical Society, Series B. 1996;**58**(1):267-288

[21] Aggarwal CC. Educational and software resources for data classification. In: Data Classification: Algorithms and Applications. 2014. pp. 657-665

[22] Batool M, Ahmad B, Choi S. A structure-based drug discovery paradigm. International Journal of Molecular Sciences. 2019:2443

[23] Dubourg-Felonneau G, Kussad Y, Kirkham D, Cassidy JW, Patel N, Clifford HW. Flatsomatic: A method for compression of somatic mutation profiles in cancer. Mach Learn Heal [Internet]. 27 November 2019;**2**(1):13-20. Available from: http://arxiv.org/abs/1911.13259 [cited: 23 February 2020]

[24] Lecun Y, Bengio Y, Hinton G. Deep learning. Nature. 2015;**521**:436-444

[25] Dubourg-Felonneau G, Darwish O, Parsons C, Rebergen D, Cassidy JW, Patel N, et al. Safety and robustness in decision making: Deep Bayesian recurrent neural networks for somatic variant calling in cancer. Mach Learn Heal [Internet]. 06 December 2019;**2**(3):31-40. Available from: http://arxiv.org/abs/1912.04174 [cited: 23 February 2020]

[26] Sanger F, Air GM, Barrell BG, Brown NL, Coulson AR, Fiddes JC, et al. Nucleotide sequence of bacteriophage φx174 DNA. Nature. 1977;**34**(2):243

[27] Craig Venter J, Adams MD, Myers EW, Li PW, Mural RJ, Sutton GG, et al. The sequence of the human genome. Science. 2001;**291**(5507):1304-1351

[28] England G. Genomics England and the 100,000 genomes project. Genomics England Website. 2003;**1**(April):233

[29] Cheng DT, Mitchell TN, Zehir A, Shah RH, Benayed R, Syed A, et al. Memorial sloan kettering-integrated mutation profiling of actionable cancer targets (MSK-IMPACT): A hybridization capture-based next-generation sequencing clinical assay for solid tumor molecular oncology. The Journal of Molecular Diagnostics. 2015;**17**(3):251-264

[30] Kim J, Kim JJ, Lee H. An analysis of disease-gene relationship from Medline abstracts by DigSee. Scientific Reports. 2017;**55**(356):5568

[31] Costa PR, Acencio ML, Lemke N. A machine learning approach for genome-wide prediction of morbid and druggable human genes based on systems-level data. BMC Genomics. 2010;**65**(5):3567

[32] Jeon J, Nim S, Teyra J, Datti A, Wrana JL, Sidhu SS, et al. A systematic approach to identify novel cancer drug targets using machine learning, inhibitor design and high-throughput screening. Genome Medicine. 2014;**23**(2):6436

[33] Ament SA, Pearl JR, Cantle JP, Bragg RM, Skene PJ, Coffey SR, et al. Transcriptional regulatory networks underlying gene expression changes in Huntington's disease. Molecular Systems Biology. 2018;**6**(3):35

[34] Rifaioglu AS, Atas H, Martin MJ, Cetin-Atalay R, Atalay V, Doğan T. Recent applications of deep learning and machine intelligence on in silico drug discovery: Methods, tools and databases. Briefings in Bioinformatics. 2019:366

[35] Mamoshina P, Volosnikova M, Ozerov IV, Putin E, Skibina E, Cortese F, et al. Machine learning on human muscle transcriptomic data for biomarker discovery and tissue-specific drug target identification. Frontiers in Genetics. 2018;**6**(3):56

[36] Lonsdale J, Thomas J, Salvatore M, Phillips R, Lo E, Shad S, et al. The genotype-tissue expression (GTEx) project. Nature Genetics. 2013;**45**:580-585

[37] Aristotelous T, Ahn S, Shukla AK, Gawron S, Sassano MF, Kahsai AW, et al. Discovery of β2 adrenergic receptor ligands using biosensor fragment screening of tagged wild-type receptor. ACS Medica Chemistry Letters [Internet]. 10 October 2013;**4**(10): 1005-1010. Available from: https://pubmed.ncbi.nlm.nih.gov/24454993

[38] Cassidy JW, Batra AS, Greenwood W, Bruna A. Patient-derived tumour xenografts for breast cancer drug discovery. Endocrine-Related Cancer. 2016:5555

[39] Zanella F, Lorens JB, Link W. High content screening: Seeing is believing. Trends in Biotechnology. 2010:234-254

[40] Fischer B, Sandmann T, Horn T, Billmann M, Chaudhary V, Huber W, et al. A map of directional genetic interactions in a metazoan cell. eLife. 2015;**1**(22):243

[41] Breinig M, Klein FA, Huber W, Boutros M. A chemical–genetic interaction map of small molecules using high-throughput imaging in cancer cells. Molecular Systems Biology. 2015;**1**(2):765-798

[42] Perlman ZE, Slack MD, Feng Y, Mitchison TJ, Wu LF, Altschuler SJ. Multidimensional drug profiling by automated microscopy. Science. 2004;**4**(1):54-65

[43] Young DW, Bender A, Hoyt J, McWhinnie E, Chirn GW, Tao CY, et al. Integrating high-content screening and ligand-target prediction to identify mechanism of action. Nature Chemical Biology. 2008;**2**(1):567-598

[44] Reisen F, Sauty De Chalon A, Pfeifer M, Zhang X, Gabriel D, Selzer P. Linking phenotypes and modes of action through high-content screen fingerprints. Assay and Drug Development Technologies. 2015;**23**(2):154

[45] Zhou XE, Melcher K, Xu HE. Understanding the GPCR biased signaling through G protein and arrestin complex structures. Current Opinion in Structural Biology. 2017;**45**:150-159

[46] Steele CW, Karim SA, Leach JDG, Bailey P, Upstill-Goddard R, Rishi L, et al. CXCR2 inhibition profoundly suppresses metastases and augments immunotherapy in pancreatic ductal adenocarcinoma. Cancer Cell. 2016;**29**(6):832-845

[47] Eash KJ, Greenbaum AM, Gopalan PK, Link DC. CXCR2 and CXCR4 antagonistically regulate neutrophil trafficking from murine bone marrow. The Journal of Clinical Investigation. 2010;**120**(7):2423-2431

[48] Tomas A, Futter CE, Eden ER. EGF receptor trafficking: Consequences for signaling and cancer. Trends in Cell Biology. 2014;**24**:26-34

[49] Guo G, Gong K, Wohlfeld B, Hatanpaa KJ, Zhao D, Habib AA. Ligand-independent EGFR signaling. Cancer Research. 2015

[50] Russell SJ, Peng KW, Bell JC. Oncolytic virotherapy. Nature Biotechnology. 2012;**30**:658-670

[51] Boltz A, Piater B, Toleikis L, Guenther R, Kolmar H, Hock B. Bi-specific aptamers mediating tumor cell lysis. The Journal of Biological Chemistry. 2011;**286**(24):21896-21905

[52] Wang J, Bardelli M, Espinosa DA, Pedotti M, Ng TS, Bianchi S, et al. A human bi-specific antibody against Zika virus with high therapeutic potential. Cell. 2017;**171**(1):229-241.e15

[53] Lounnas V, Ritschel T, Kelder J, McGuire R, Bywater RP, Foloppe N. Current progress in structure-based rational drug design marks a new mindset in drug discovery. Computational and Structural Biotechnology Journal. 2013;**5**:e201302011

[54] Kalyaanamoorthy S, Chen YPP. Structure-based drug design to augment hit discovery. Drug Discovery Today. 2011;**16**:831-839

[55] Laurie ATR, Jackson RM. Q-SiteFinder: An energy-based method for the prediction of protein-ligand binding sites. Bioinformatics. 2005;**21**(9):1908-1916

[56] Nayal M, Honig B. On the nature of cavities on protein surfaces: Application to the identification of drug-binding sites. Proteins: Structure, Function, and Genetics. 2006;**65**(3):568

[57] McMillan EA, Ryu MJ, Diep CH, Mendiratta S, Clemenceau JR, Vaden RM, et al. Chemistry-first approach for nomination of personalized treatment in lung cancer. Cell. 2018;**86**(5):356

[58] Ramsundar B, Liu B, Wu Z, Verras A, Tudor M, Sheridan RP, et al. Is multitask deep learning practical for pharma? Journal of Chemical Information and Modeling. 2017;**57**(8):2068-2076

[59] Wu Z, Ramsundar B, Feinberg EN, Gomes J, Geniesse C, Pappu AS, et al. MoleculeNet: A benchmark for molecular machine learning. Chemical Science. 2018;**9**(3):367

[60] Altae-Tran H, Ramsundar B, Pappu AS, Pande V. Low data drug discovery with one-shot learning. ACS Central Science. 2017;**3**(4):283-293

[61] Barati Farimani A, Feinberg E, Pande V. Binding pathway of opiates to μ-opioid receptors revealed by machine learning. Biophysical Journal. 2018;**76**(3):677

[62] Ma J, Sheridan RP, Liaw A, Dahl GE, Svetnik V. Deep neural nets as a method for quantitative structure-activity relationships. Journal of Chemical Information and Modeling. 2015;**55**(2):263-274

[63] Mayr A, Klambauer G, Unterthiner T, Hochreiter S. DeepTox: Toxicity prediction using deep learning. Frontiers in Environmental Science. 2016;**3**(FEB):231-123

[64] Kadurin A, Nikolenko S, Khrabrov K, Aliper A, Zhavoronkov A. DruGAN: An advanced generative adversarial autoencoder model for de novo generation of new molecules with desired molecular properties in silico. Molecular Pharmaceutics. 2017;**14**(9):3098-3104

[65] Zhao K, So H-C. A machine learning approach to drug repositioning based on drug expression profiles: Applications to schizophrenia and depression/anxiety disorders. bioRxiv [Internet]. Available from: https://arxiv.org/pdf/1706.03014.pdf

[66] Musa A, Ghoraie LS, Zhang SD, Glazko G, Yli-Harja O, Dehmer M, et al. A review of connectivity map and computational approaches in pharmacogenomics. Briefings in Bioinformatics. 2018;**34**(3):254-267

Section 2

Structuring Data

Chapter 3

Dimensionality and Structure in Cancer Genomics: A Statistical Learning Perspective

Jacob Bradley

Abstract

Computational analysis of genomic data has transformed research and clinical practice in oncology. Machine learning and AI advancements hold promise for answering theoretical and practical questions. While the modern researcher has access to a catalogue of tools from disciplines such as natural language processing and image recognition, before browsing for our favourite off-the-shelf technique it is worth asking a sequence of questions. What sort of data are we dealing with in cancer genomics? Do we have enough of it to be successful without designing into our models what we already know about its structure? If our methods do work, will we understand why? Are our tools robust enough to be applied in clinical practice? If so, are the technologies upon which they rely economically viable? While we will not answer all of these questions, we will provide language with which to discuss them. Understanding how much information we can expect to extract from data is a statistical question.

Keywords: dimensionality, sparsity, high-dimensional statistics, cancer genomics, biomarkers, learning theory

1. Introduction

This chapter should be equally approachable to those with a background in machine learning/statistics and those with a more biological background. Beginning with a contextualisation of cancer genomics as the starting point for drug and biomarker discovery, we will attempt to convince the reader that statistical theory serves as the backbone and language of modern developments in machine learning. In order to facilitate those with less experience in biology, we will provide a very brief introduction to the types of data encountered in sequencing-based studies and the opportunities and problems they present. After providing some terminology and useful concepts from high-dimensional statistics, we will discuss how these concepts arise naturally in the context of cancer genomics, with some illustrative examples of how different techniques may be employed in translational scientific research. We will conclude by providing sketches of some modern developments and a description of the transition from what can loosely be termed statistical learning to what nowadays is referred to as machine learning.

1.1 Cancer genomics in drug discovery

Since the success of the Human Genome Project [1], sequencing technologies have improved at an exponential rate, both in terms of cost per megabase sequenced and the number of individuals who have had some portion of their genome sequenced (although the cost remains higher in practice than often reported) [2]. This has introduced an invaluable new resource for biomedical research in general. For the study of cancer, a disease of the genome, the ability to rapidly and cheaply sequence normal and tumour-derived DNA has transformed basic research, birthing the field of cancer genomics. This is beginning to impact frontline clinical oncology [3]. Whole genome sequencing is not yet standard of care for the generic cancer patient, but access to in-depth genetic data is becoming more common. Initiatives such as the 10,000/100,000 Genomes Projects [4] and The Cancer Genome Atlas [5] have given researchers access to large clinical datasets with a variety of accompanying omics data.

Understanding the genomic landscape of cancer genomes is critical to the drug discovery pipeline [6], particularly in pre-clinical identification of targets and biomarkers. Knowledge of the location and associated products of oncogenes (genes in which mutation can cause a cell to become cancerous) can allow for intelligent selection of druggable sites and identification of tumour suppressor genes (genes that under normal circumstances prevent uncontrolled cell division) gives options for therapies which may replace patients' defective cell cycle control mechanisms. Alongside new drugs, it is becoming increasingly common for therapies to be offered alongisde genomic biomarkers, which may stratify patients who are more likely to benefit from the treatment [7, 8].

These new sources and types of data allow researchers a greatly expanded toolbox with which to investigate the causes and development of cancer, but also present a unique set of challenges. The number of covaraiates in omics datasets causes a variety of theoretical and practical problems for classical statistical analysis, a problem often referred to as the curse of dimensionality [9].

1.2 Statistical learning and machine learning

Informally, the field of high-dimensional statistics attempts to address theoretical and computational problems associated with datasets in which the number of covariates (in our case this may refer to chromosomal locations or genes) is comparable to or greater than the number of samples available. In these settings results such as the central limit theorem that rely on divergence of the sample size independent of the dimensionality are often not of much use [10]. This is often the case in cancer genomics.

Recent decades have seen much excitement around the application of machine learning methods to a wide variety of high-dimensional problems. Particular progress has been made in automated image recognition and natural language processing (NLP). This progress has come via the development of specialised techniques to exploit the **structure** inherent in each data type (e.g. convolutional neural networks for image recognition [11] and word embedding for NLP [12]), but also from a vastly increased pool of data on which to train models. These data resources have typically been collected online, where there exists an abundance of labelled and unlabelled images and pieces of text.

It is hoped that similar strides forward can be anticipated in biology, but it is important to acknowledge the current gap in data availability between cancer genomics and the other machine learning disciplines mentioned above. In the next section we will discuss typical types of biological data encountered in cancer genomics (including sequencing-based omics technologics that may not strictly be genomics, such as gene expression profiling), their dimensionality and typical availability. While efforts to deploy machine learning architectures are certainly producing results in some cases [13, 14], an important takeaway is that in many cases, we are not yet in a situation where the data-heavy deep learning approaches that have revolutionised image recognition will be applicable to cancer genomics problems.

That is not to say that we cannot do anything! In fact, it is often instructive to try and make headway in situations where a 'data-heavy, structure-light' approach is unsuitable, and these sorts of investigations can have a profound impact on the design of more sophisticated models [15]. As a final point, readers approaching without a significant backlog of machine learning expertise will find that an understanding of statistical terminology will aid comprehension of the machine learning literature which has them as its basis.

2. Omics and biological data

2.1 DNA sequencing

Cancer genomics is underpinned by the ability to sequence DNA cheaply and quickly. DNA is organised into chromosomes, along each of which many genes are arranged, with further non-coding regions interspersed in-between. The fundamental units of DNA are nucleotide bases, of which there are four varieties (labelled C, G, T and A). These are organised in groups of length three called codons, which code for the production amino acids. Codons are arranged in sequences such that their amino acids when joined in chain form proteins—the products of genes.

The aim of sequencing is to read, base by base, the information content of DNA. This was originally done by Sanger sequencing, a procedure to infer the base composition of a piece of DNA one base at a time. High-throughput sequencing automates this process via the following workflow:

1. DNA is isolated from a sample and amplified (replicated many times) to ensure good signal.

2. Purified DNA is broken into many pieces of manageable length.

3. These short strands are sequenced individually and simultaneously by an automated process similar to Sanger sequencing.

4. These short sequences are matched to a reference human genome to identify where the DNA in the original sample differed from that reference.

2.1.1 Tumour/normal variants

In cancer, some subset of cells accumulate mutations, via random misreplication of DNA during cell division or exposure to some external mutagen (e.g. cigarette smoke, UV light). Tumour cells therefore contain DNA with a different sequence to that of the patients' typical sequence. To understand this two samples are collected, one from the tumour and one from normal tissue, and both are sequenced. The sequences are compared and this produces a list of locations at which mutations have occured: these mutations can have a variety of types (replacements, insertions, etc.) and can have vastly differing functional implications.

In simplest setting, we could express a tumour's mutational profile as a vector, with each component corresponding to whether the tumour-derived and normal sequences match at that point. How long would this vector be? The human genome contains approximately 3×10^9 base locations. This is the dimensionality (which we will refer to later on as p) of naively presented genomic data. We often like to compare the dimensionality of a dataset with the number of samples (which we will later call n) to which we can expect to have access. In this case, unless we have access to tumour profiling for more than a third of all humans on the planet, we can never hope that these numbers will be comparable. We could make a small gain by listing all codons in the genome, labelling a component as one if the codon has been functionally altered by mutations and zero otherwise. Here though we would still have $p = 10^9$.

We could simplify our data further. Decades of biological research has focused on cataloguing the locations of genes across the genome. We might consider as covariates each of the (approximately 2×10^4) genes, and represent each sample as a vector where each component refers to (a) whether or not the gene contained a functional mutation; (b) how many such mutations were present; or (c) some other representation of the severity of collective mutations presents in the gene, drawing upon known biology. It is important to appreciate the trade-off we have made here: we have imposed an external notion of structure onto our data and in return have greatly reduced the dimensionality (by five orders of magnitude), but in exchange have lost resolution and thus potential information. This gain/sacrifice will be reflected when we choose to make even further structural assumptions in order to construct sensible models.

2.1.2 Heterogeneity and depth

Another important concern for those dealing with cancer genome data is that tumours are often highly heterogeneous. Different sub-populations of cells have different mutation profiles, which fit into an evolutionary hierarchy within the tumour's history. The importance of understanding the role of heterogeneity is beginning to be appreciated in a clinical context, and this has implications for the type of data that are used. In the context of the high-throughput sequencing pipeline, the relevant quantity is depth: identifying not just one but a variety of tumour sequences at a genomic locus along with the proportion in which they occur means thinking very hard about how best to express that data.

2.2 Gene expression

It is often not just the sequence of a gene which it relevant in a tumour, but the level of gene expression. The way that this is most often estimated is via the proxy of RNA transcript abundance: RNA is a similar molecule to DNA that is produced during the process of DNA being 'read', and acts as a messenger for sequences that should be converted to protein. Abundances of different RNA transcripts can be measured using procedures based on DNA sequencing. This will in general give data with the same dimensionality as gene-based mutation data, but is of a different type. Measured values are continuous to represent concentrations of gene products, rather than discrete 'mutated/not mutated' values. This has implications as to the sort of structural assumptions we can make about the data that we observe, and the models that will be best suited to capitalise on that structure.

DOI: http://dx.doi.org/10.5772/intechopen.92574

3. Dimensionality and structure in statistical learning theory

Now familiar with the most relevant biological concepts, we turn to the mathematical theory of high-dimensional statistics, which has experienced a surge of interest in the last two decades. This is the language with which we will be attempting to interrogate issues of inference and prediction in cancer genomics. Informally, we may think of high-dimensional statistics to be concerned with the realm in which the dimensionality of our input data, p, is comparable to or greater than the number of training samples n we have available. In this regime the classical asymptotic theory of statistics, which generally relies on an assumption of fixed dimension and considers limiting behaviour as $n \to \infty$, may fail to apply. Classical results such as the law of large numbers and central limit theorem are not applicable.

3.1 What is high-dimensional statistics?

We often consider a very generic setup, in which we have paired data $\{(x_1,y_1),(x_2,y_2),\dots,(x_n,y_n)\}$. We model each of these pairs as being drawn from a joint probability distribution $P_{X\times Y}$, which gives the probability of observing any combination of observation x and label y. For now we make no assumptions about the nature of the y_i labels: they may be continuous values (regression), discrete values (classification) or more complicated objects such as is the case in survival analysis. We assume that $x_i \in \mathcal{X} \subset \mathbb{R}^p$ for each $1 \le i \le n$, so that our observed values are vectors of length p and each element is a real number (possibly restricted to some subset such as the positive reals—this is what $\mathcal{X}$ specifies). We refer to p as the dimension and n as the sample size of our data. We wish to fit some model $\mathcal{M}$ to the data. This could be in order to make some inference about the parameters of the distribution $P_{X\times Y}$, which will hopefuly shed light on the effect of each of the covariates contained in an observation x. Alternatively, we might be trying to predict future values of y from unlabelled observations as accurately as possible. These two aims are often distinguished by the umbrella terms statistical inference and statistical learning.

In many statistical models we have a vector β of parameters with at least the same dimension as our data ($\beta \in \mathbb{R}^q,\ q \ge p$). In generalised linear models (GLMs) the likelihood of an observation y depends upon the data x_i solely via the inner product $x_i^T\beta$, so that each component of β corresponds to the relative importance of its associated covariate. Classically, we would attempt to to estimate the parameter β via our observation through a procedure such as likelihood maximisation. However, it is clear in this context that if p is comparable to or larger than n then we have very little chance of accurately inferring the parameter vector β. For example, we canot expect to simultaneously learn about the effect of 20 covariates if we only have 10 observations: we say here that the model is unidentifiable.

High-dimensional statistics attempts to gauge what we can do in regimes such as these. One is approach is to assume the data has some low-dimensional structure. This means that we can embed our data in a lower dimensional space such that the smaller representation of our data contains all or most of the necessary information about the joint distribution $P_{X\times Y}$. We will discuss some common structural assumptions. The simplest and most interpretable is sparsity.

Definition 3.1. (Sparsity): 'Relatively few covariates are important'.

Given a vector $\beta \in \mathbb{R}^p$ parameterising a model, we say β is k-sparse, for $k \le p$, if at most k elements of β are non-zero, that is

$$|\beta|_0 := \sum_{j=1}^{p} \mathbf{1}\{\beta_j \neq 0\} \leq k.$$

We can say a model $\mathcal{M}$ parameterised by a vector β is k-sparse if the vector β is k-sparse.

Sparsity is a useful assumption to make for a variety of reasons. We are reducing the number of parameters that we must estimate—for a k-sparse model, we need only estimate k parameters. Before we do so we need to decide which k parameters are allowed to be non-zero, that is, to which k-dimensional subspace (out of $\binom{p}{k}$ choices) our parameter belongs. In practice this is not a huge issue—some powerful theory from the field of convex optimisation allows for efficient training of sparse models (see the LASSO estimator below). Finally, sparse models are interpretable. A small number of covariates selected for importance can be useful in hypothesis refinement.

3.1.1 Sparse data vs. sparse models

It is worth at this point drawing a distinction between two phenomena in statistics and data science both referred to as 'sparsity', both of which are exhibited in cancer genomics. The first is sparse *data*, in which almost all observed data points have the same value (typically zero). Mutation data displays this trait—the rate at which mutations occur in the genome varies widely across and within cancer types, but rarely exceeds 100 Mut/Mb, that is one mutation per 10^4 nucleotide base pairs [16]. This sparsity is exploited in the way that tumour/normal DNA data is stored, in file formats such as VCF (variant called format) and MAF (mutation annotated format). Many programming languages and data science packages have data structures optimised for sparse data, and it is also often possible to optimise learning and algorithms for sparse data. However, here we will focus on sparse *models*. These are models where it is assumed that only a small subspace of the covariate space is relevant, via assumptions such as the one described above.

This notion that there is some sparse representation of data but that it may not translate directly to a subset of our covariates motivates the more general principle of Sufficient Dimension Reduction (SDR). Sparsity restricts our attention to some small subspace of the covariate space $\mathbb{R}^p$. More generally, we may insist on some important smaller subspace, but one that does not depending on a specific representation of our data x. The definition of SDR is somewhat more technical, so those without mathematical background may find it easier to skip.

Definition 3.2. (Sufficient Dimension Reduction): 'Some small representation of our data contains all the important information'.

Given (X, Y) drawn from probability distribution $P_{X \times Y}$, we say there exists a sufficient dimension reduction of size d^* if there exists some function $S : \mathbb{R}^p \to \mathbb{R}^{d^*}$ with $d^* < p$ such that Y is conditionally independent of X given $S(X)$, that is,

$$Y \perp\!\!\!\perp X \mid S(X)$$

For an observation x, the image $S(X)$ is a d^*-dimensional representation of x. As a special case we have linear sufficient dimensional reduction if the function S is a linear projection $A^* : \mathbb{R}^p \to \mathbb{R}^{d^*}$.

Picking apart this definition, conditional independence means that Y only depends on X through some low-dimensional image. Note that, in contrast to sparsity, we have not made reference to a linear model parameter β. In fact, in the context of a generalised linear model where Y depends on X only through some function of $\beta^T X$, we can simply take $S(X) = A^* X = \beta^T$ and see that Y admits a sufficient dimensionality condition with $d^* = 1$. SDR, therefore, is a helpful notion in settings in which we need to apply a non-linear model structure. Methods based on finding sufficient dimension reduction projections by searching through spaces of projections [17] in combination with non-linear base classifiers are beginning to show promise in a variety of domains including the analysis of high-dimensional medical data [18].

3.1.2 Techniques in high-dimensional statistics: Selection and regularisation

It is all very well imposing assumptions of low-dimensional structure onto our data. How can we now exploit this to produce models that reflect the structural assumptions we have made? One answer is regularisation. Regularisation refers to some penalisation process being applied to the parameters of our model. The intuition is that, given some model parameter β of size greater than or equal to the dimension p of our data, and thus of comparable magnitude to our number of samples, we have enough degrees of freedom when fitting the model that we can be guaranteed to produce almost perfect training set results without having done anything more than memorise our data. Therefore we must place restrictions on our parameter, and the trick is to do this as part of the model fitting process by combining a regularisation term to the loss function of our learning procedure (ideally in such a way as to preserve what is known as loss convexity, which allows efficient model fitting).

Regularisation is applied in practice across a whole range of model types, but is easiest to understand in the context of linear regression, so in the discussion that follows we will restrict ourselves to this setting.

In linear regression we have a model $\mathcal{M}_\beta$, parameterised by β, given by

$$\mathcal{M}_\beta : Y_i = X_i^T \beta + \varepsilon, \tag{1}$$

for some noise ε. We are saying that Y can be approximated by a linear combination of the components of X, with the relative weightings of each component given by the components of β. The loss of our model (a measure of how inaccurately it is predicting across all our data) is given by

$$\mathcal{L}(\mathcal{M}_\beta) = \frac{1}{n} \sum_{i=1}^{n} \left(Y_i - X_i^T \beta\right)^2. \tag{2}$$

In general we choose β to minimise this loss for an optimal model, but suppose we wish to find an optimal k-sparse model, that is one for which β is k-sparse. Rather than minimising over all possible choices of β, we are minimising the loss over all values of β that are also k-sparse:

$$\min_{\beta \in \mathbb{R}^p,\ |\beta|_0 \le k} \left\{ \mathcal{L}(\mathcal{M}_\beta) \right\}. \tag{3}$$

Here we face a computational difficulty: we have to separately check each subset of covariates of size k and minimise on that set of possible parameters, then compare them all to find the best. What we do to circumvent this is include a penalisation term for β, which encourages sparsity alongside the loss function in our optimisation. An obvious choice would be the L0 'norm', $|\beta|_0$, which counts non-zero coefficients. In practice this is not computationally feasible (to be technical, the problem is non-convex and so NP-hard), so instead we use the the L1 norm $|\beta|_1$

given by $\sum_{j=1}^{p}|\beta_j|$. While this does not explicitly encode sparsity, it turns out that in practice it does produce sparse solutions. This process of replacing a non-convex problem with an easier one is in general called convex relaxation.

Technique 3.1. (Regularisation for Sparsity: L1/LASSO): Given the setup above, L1 regularised estimation (known in the case of linear regression as the LASSO estimator [19]) selects β solving the following optimisation

$$\min_{\beta\in\mathbb{R}^p}\left\{\sum_{i=1}^{n}\mathcal{L}(\mathcal{M}_\beta)+\lambda|\beta|_1\right\}$$

where λ is a positive number chosen to specify how strongly we want to encourage sparsity: different values of λ will produce different k s in the ouput. A particularly attractive feature of the LASSO selector is that it acts simultaneously as a variable selection and model fitting procedure.

To take stock, we have begun with an assumption that some small subset of our covariates are important in predicting the response Y. This assumption might have come from necessity due to data availability, from knowledge of the biological system we are modelling, or from both. We will discuss these possibilities in more depth in the next chapter. We have taken a simple model, and altered it to express this structure, and have done so in a way that is computationally feasible.

The specific form of the regularisation we employ can have very subtle effects on the traits it encourages in models, which should motivate us to be very careful when translating the biological knowledge we want to express into our learning systems. For example, adding an identical regularisation term but replacing the L1 norm with the L2 norm ($|\beta|_2=\sqrt{\sum\beta_i^2}$) does not produce sparse models, but rather models that do not contain large coefficients. The corresponding structural assumption for this is slightly more technical (we can assert a multivariate Gaussian prior on the parameter space for β). This can be applied in a wide variety of high-dimensional situations, often alongside other forms of regularisation, as a combatant to over-fitting (typically via cross-validation).

Technique 3.2. (Regularisation for Dimension: L2/Ridge Regression): L2 regularised estimation (known as ridge regression in the linear setting [19]) selects β solving the following optimisation

$$\min_{\beta\in\mathbb{R}^p}\left\{\sum_{i=1}^{n}\mathcal{L}(\mathcal{M}_\beta)+\lambda|\beta|_2\right\}$$

where again λ is a positive value that can be selected by cross-validation to reduce overfitting.

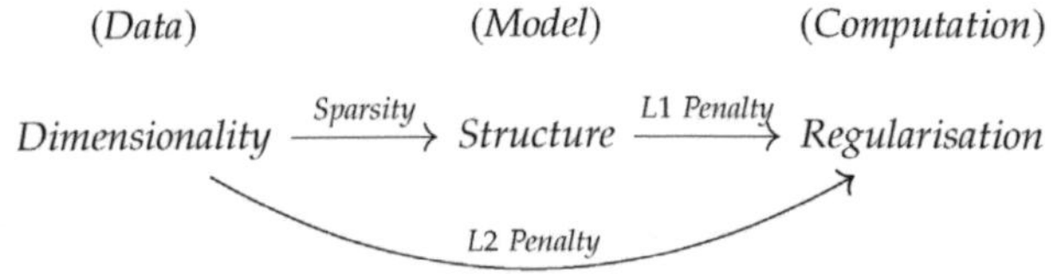

Figure 1.
An example of a high-dimensional workflow, where high dimensionality is addressed via the imposition of model structure, in this case sparsity. This is translated into a computationally tractable extension of standard regression model fitting via an L1 penalty. Dimension-induced overfitting is simultaneously managed via L2 regularisation. If sparsity is a reasonable structural assumption, that is few covariates have genuine impact, L2 regularisation should have a relatively small impact.

Figure 1 describes the workflow of modelling high-dimensional data. The data dimensionality, as discussed in the previous chapter, is the underlying problem, which we address with structural assumptions informed from a mixture of external knowledge and practicality, which are then transformed into a feasible computational problem. Intuition around the biological and also statistical context are applied at each step.

For those unsatisfied with the abstract nature of the discussion above, we now attempt to provide more concrete examples.

4. Cancer genomics questions in the language of high-dimensional statistics

4.1 Biomarker/driver gene identification

We have discussed some of the terminology associated with high-dimensional statistics. We can now express some cancer genomics questions in the same language. We have data with a very high dimensionality p: bases, codons or genes ($p \approx 3 \times 10^9$, 1×10^9 and 2×10^4 respectively) and we would like to predict some outcome, be it a survival value, biomarker signature or other phenotype. Due to the resources and time required to perform whole genome or exome sequencing we often face restrictions in the number of samples at our disposal. The popular Cancer Genome Atlas resource [5], for example, contains sequencing data for around 20,000 tumour/normal matched samples. Even if all of these samples were relevant to our study, and we were trying to predict some phenotype Y using gene-level data, we would be working in the $p \approx n$ regime. If we were using codon or nucleotide level information, we would be well into the $p > > n$ regime. In the following we will assume we are working with some gene-level covariates, and investigate what sort of structural assumptions we may wish to make in order to fit tractable and robust models.

4.2 Sparsity by assumption: driver genes

Driver genes in the simplest sense are genes that, when mutated, will elevate risk of the development, progression or adaptation of a tumour [20]. They may be grouped roughly into oncogenes and tumour suppressors: oncogenes admit mutations giving some selective advantage to a cancer cell, while tumour suppressors in their standard form protect against aberrant cell growth or apoptosis evasion. Identifying driver genes (or driver sites within genes) among the extensive backdrop mutation in tumours is notoriously difficult. Selection pressures produce subtle and often non-obvious patterns of mutation density between neutral and non-neutral genes as well as distinct signatures for oncogenes and tumour suppressors [21]. Neglecting these difficulties for now, suppose we wish to infer some phenotype Y (again for simplicity we assume that this is continuous and single-valued). We do not have nearly enough data to fully explore the dependence of Y on all genes simultaneously—we have to assume that there are *relatively few relevant features/driver genes*. This is exactly a sparsity assumption—a regularisation method such as LASSO might be helpful. The advantages of this are twofold. We have identified a set of genes of interest, which might form the basis for some targeted prognostic panel, while simultaneously inferring a predictive structure on top of this list of genes. The added interpretability of our model given by assuming a structural restraint is useful when verifying our results in the lab. We have produced a manageable set of interesting genes that can be investigated on a more detailed individual basis.

4.3 Sparsity by necessity: gene panels for genome-wide biomarkers

Another justification for selecting some small set of genes/genomic loci to include in an investigative panel is that the cost and time to perform sequencing depends (approximately linearly) on the size of the subsection of the genome to be sequenced, and the depth at which it is sequenced. This means that in many practical or clinical environments, cost is a major factor. While the cost of whole genome sequencing has decreased at an impressive rate, it is far from being standard of care for cancer patients. It is therefore important that gene-panel style biomarkers are as small as possible, while maintaining enough accuracy that clinicians feel confident in acting upon predictions. This is a particular issue for genome-wide biomarkers, which have gained popularity in recent years, for example in cancer immunotherapy. Examples include tumour mutation burden [22] and indel burden [23], which report density of somatic mutation across the entire cancer genome. In this case all regions of the genome are relevant to greater or lesser extent (**Figure 2**)—the optimal panel for prediction would be the entire genome (or exome, depending on the specific biomarker). However, certain genes may be particularly relevant, for example by taking an active role in DNA repair mechanisms. When estimating such biomarkers, we therefore want to offset the positive predictive contributions of individual genes/loci against the added cost burden given by inclusion in the panel. Analyses of the impact of panel size on predictive power in theoretical and practical settings are becoming more common [24].

Suppose we have some set G of genes, where g refers to an individual gene with coding sequence of length n_g. Now let $P \subset G$ refer to a gene panel comprising a set of genes, and $\mathcal{M}_P$ be a model trained on some data with covariates included according to the gene panel P. Then we might wish to solve the optimisation problem

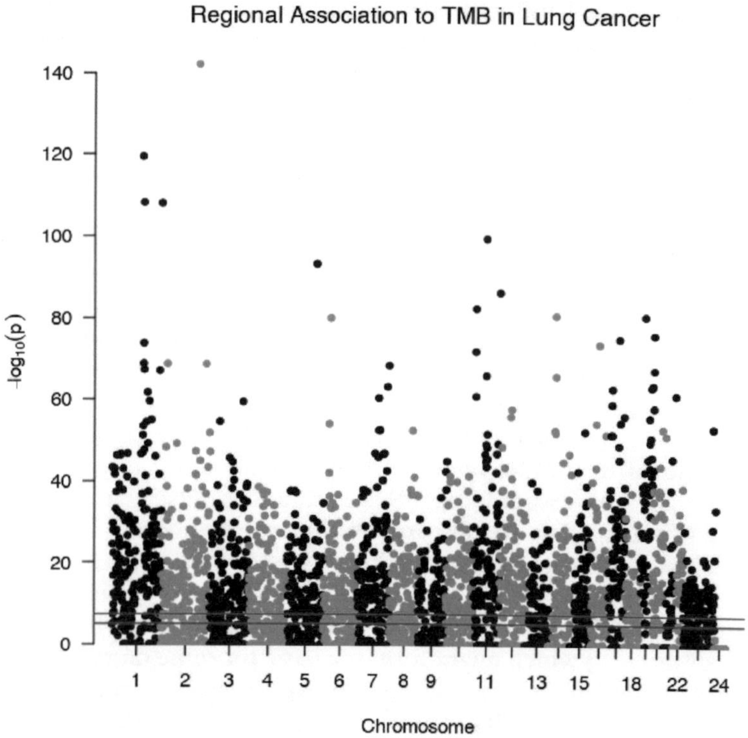

Figure 2.
For an additive, genome-wide biomarker such as TMB (tumour mutational burden), all genomic loci are significantly correlated with TMB (unlike in typical GWAS studies). How do we choose a subset that is not prohibitively large but can reliably estimate the marker via some predictive model?

$$\min_{P \subset G} \{\mathcal{L}(\mathcal{M}_P)\} \quad \text{such that} \quad |P| \leq L, \tag{4}$$

where $\mathcal{L}(\mathcal{M})$ is the loss of the model $\mathcal{M}$, $|P| = \sum_{g \in P} n_g$ is the total length of the gene panel P and L is some prescribed maximum panel length. Note the similarity with the LASSO setup described in Section 3.1. In the case of a linear model we can similarly reformulate the problem in terms of the parameter β, and solve the analogous problem.

Technique 4.1. (Weighted L1 Regularisation/LASSO): Here we select β satisfying the optimisation problem

$$\min_{\beta \in \mathbb{R}^{|G|}} \left\{ \mathcal{L}(\mathcal{M}_\beta) + \lambda \sum_{g \in G} n_g |\beta_g| \right\}$$

where we have again swapped the panel length bound L for the regularisation parameter λ. Since all the n_g values are positive, this is still a convex optimisation problem and thus can be solved efficiency as in the standard case. Choice of λ is less likely to be chosen via cross-fitting, as smaller values of λ will always improve predictive power. Instead λ will be chosen to control the size of the resulting gene panel.

4.3.1 Distinguishing causative mutations

It should again be noted that these are illustrations of how high-dimensional model construction is done. In reality many more subtleties may have to be taken into account. In the above a key caveat requiring understanding is the role of selective pressure in cancer-relevant genes [25], and how this affects the mutation rate in different sections of the genome [26]. One way this can be investigated is by looking at the relative predictive power of synonymous and non-synonymous mutations for genome-wide mutation burden [27]. The gold standard for identifying causative relationships between genotype and phenotype, however, remains with functional validation studies.

4.4 Survival prediction

No review of statistical learning in cancer genomics would be complete without a mention of survival prediction. Survival prediction is useful in a variety of situations, far beyond direct prognostic application. Hazard regression models based on genomic data have been useful in identifying therapeutic resistance [28] or general prognosis [29, 30] factors, which are of great interest to those developing drugs or attempting to understand which patients can expect to benefit from them. Regularisation-based techniques are perfectly adaptable to proportional-hazards style models [31], to which end there has much literature beyond what we have scope to discuss in this chapter.

5. Modern techniques in high-dimensional statistics and dimensionality reduction

We conclude with some examples from recent literature of techniques related to dimensionality reduction in modelling genomic data. The examples have been chosen to demonstrate the structure/regularisation workflow discussed in this chapter, and are small a set of examples rather than (anywhere near) an exhaustive list.

5.1 Regularised graphical models

In the regression examples discussed previously, the parameters of interest have represented the weighted effect of observed covariates on a label. In supervised and unsupervised cases, we are also often interesting in looking at how closely related different covariates are, through estimating the correlation matrix of the observation variable X. If we have an observation of dimensionality p, then the covariance matrix will be of size p^2, so problems of estimation from small n are even more confounded!

Two forms of regularisation are popular, often used in tandem. The first is a sparsity penalty applied to all matrix entries [32]. What does this correspond to structurally? It means that that most pairs of covariates are independent (or at least uncorrelated). This is a very relevant notion in network analysis, where variables are thought to affect each other in a way that can be described by some graphical structure. Sparsity of matrix elements then corresponds to sparsity of the graph describing the network. It is also not uncommon to sparsely penalise precision, defined by the components of the inverse covariance matrix [33].

Alternately (or in addition), we may wish to limit the number of distinct *patterns* of correlation, so that all covariates display a correlation profile that is made up of a combination of a relatively small set of base signatures. This structure may be fitted for by imposing rank-based regularisation [34, 35]. For those wanting a greater appreciation of the theory, the way this is imposed is another good example of convex penalty relaxation (as was achieved by switching from the L_0 to L_1 norm in sparsity regularisation), where here the nuclear norm is used as the convex relaxation of matrix rank.

5.2 Localised sparsity assumptions

We have made an extensive discussion of sparse models in this chapter. We might wonder if there are any generalisations to the assumption that relatively few of our covariates are important throughout all of our samples. One such generalisation would be that for some subsets of our samples sparsity assumptions hold, but that the important covariates may differ from subset to subset within our data. In a localised sparsity setting, we are often given some knowledge of the organisational structure of data, either in a discrete way through a prior partition of the samples or network structure, or in a continuous way through a measure of distance between samples (which may come directly from the input data). We can then fit linear models that are regularised towards sparsity, but where variable selection is allowed to vary between samples, and allowed to vary more between samples that are more distant. This has been applied to the prediction of drug toxicity based on differential gene expression data [36].

5.3 Variational autoencoders

For our final example we consider a notion of dimensionality reduction that is more general and that has been studied extensively in the machine learning literature. This nicely elucidates the grey border between statistical and machine learning, and the difficulties and opportunities available to biological research by embracing the latter.

Variational autoencoders (VAEs) are a class of neural networks with a variety of architectures and sizes, but whose premise centres around producing an encoding/decoding framework between high-dimensional data and a lower dimensional

DOI: http://dx.doi.org/10.5772/intechopen.92574

representation [37]. VAEs have an 'hourglass' shape: input data is fed into the network, and information is propagated through layers of progressively smaller size until a bottleneck is reached. The central layer will have some small number of latent nodes. Subsequent layers increase in size, reaching an output of dimension matching the input. VAEs are trained to reproduce the inputs with which they are trained as accurately as possible. We can then view the central latent nodes as an encoding of our input data [38]. This might (a) contain some insightful information and (b) be useful as lower dimensional input data for training other models.

In the context of cancer genomics [39], VAEs pose two challenges, illustrative of those that machine learning procedures in general must overcome to be useful in a basic research or clinical setting. Firstly, they are highly parameterised compared to the types of model discussed so far. We have discussed at length the balance between data availability and model size, and the significant extra effort necessary to extract information when information is scarce. One of the advantages of deep learning procedures is their versatility and lack of dependence on prior knowledge and assumptions of structure. The cost is that they are very data intensive, prohibitively so in some cases. Secondly, while a VAE's latent nodes may be informative within a network, there is no necessary guarantee that they will be interpretable by a human, nor that biologically relevant features will have been neatly allocated to a single node. Strategies to 'untangle' VAEs are necessary to make biologically relevant predictions [40].

6. Conclusions

The dimensionality of data in genomics is a sticking point that at its full potency is more debilitating than in any other research discipline [9]. Even at the current pace of increase of the availability of sequencing data, it will be a long time away (if ever) that the most powerful and general machine learning techniques will be at our disposal without recourse to the vast wealth of biological knowledge we as a species have accumulated. To properly use that knowledge, we need researchers who are able to speak the language of both camps. It is not sufficient that researchers in cancer genomics provide data and questions to researchers in machine learning, nor that machine learning researchers communicate back the output of their methods. Instead, methods need to be crafted bespokely by those who understand what features of cancer data are relevant, how those features manifest themselves and how to exploit them in a mathematically consistent way.

This entire workflow is quite easy to follow when the sort of structure we are insisting upon in our models is very simple. Even when a structural assumption can be motivated in a single sentence (see Definition 3.1), and a model is simple (such as in linear regression), a good design of learning procedure might not be immediately obvious. It can likely, however, be given a fairly ground-up description within a single book chapter. When the structural assumptions we really want to incorporate might well extend as far as our current appreciation of the mutational processes affecting tumours across heterogenuous cell populations, chromosomes, genes and codons, and the models we want to fit are similarly at the cutting edge of computational research, then the position of an interdisciplinary researcher may well require far more legwork to maintain.

As motivation for the above legwork, it should go without saying that cancer genomics in the machine learning age has potential to do a great deal of good in the long term. Yet uncovering a deeper understanding of how cancer works is not the only worthwhile goal. Designing procedures that can work *now* to be more effective, sometimes crossing a threshold between non-pracitcality and practicality (in some part of the world), can have a more immediate benefit. In the clinic, the time scale and cost of data collection are not abstract mathematical problems, so designing a test that works with less data can be just as enabling as uncovering a new paradigm of cancer progression.

Acknowledgements

Many thanks to Timothy Cannings and Belle Taylor for their support and advice, to John Cassidy for suggestions of improvements, to Steven Bradley for proofreading and providing a non-technical reader's viewpoint, and to Morton for his invaluable contributions.

Conflict of interest

The author declares no conflict of interests.

Author details

Jacob Bradley[1,2]

1 School of Mathematics, University of Edinburgh, UK

2 Cambridge Cancer Genomics, Cambridge, UK

*Address all correspondence to: j.r.j.bradley@ed.ac.uk.com

References

[1] Lander E, Chen C, Linton L, Birren B, Nusbaum C, Zody M, et al. Initial sequencing and analysis of the human genome. Nature. 2001;**409**:860-921

[2] Sboner A, Xinmeng M, Greenbaum D, Auerbach R, Gerstein M. The real cost of sequencing: Higher than you think! Genome Biology. 2011;**12**:125

[3] Prokop J, May T, Strong K, Bilinovich S, Bupp C, Rajasekaran S, et al. Genome sequencing in the clinic: The past, present, and future of genomic medicine. Physiological Genomics. 2018;**50**:563-579

[4] Telenti A, Pierce L, Biggs W, di Iulio J, Wong E, Fabani M, et al. Deep sequencing of 10,000 human genomes. Proceedings of the National Academy of Sciences. 2016;**113**:11901-11906

[5] Weinstein JN, Collisson EA, Mills GB. The cancer genome atlas pan-cancer analysis project. Nature Genetics. 2013;**45**(10):1113-1120

[6] Raja R, Lee Y, Streicher K, Conway J, Wu S, Sridhar S, et al. Integrating genomics into drug discovery and development: Challenges and aspirations. Pharmaceutical Medicine. 2017;**31**: 217-233

[7] Weber B, Hager H, Sorensen B, Mcculloch T, Mellemgaard A, Khalil A, et al. EGFR mutation frequency and effectiveness of erlotinib: A prospective observational study in Danish patients with non-small cell lung cancer. Lung Cancer. 2013;**83**:224-230

[8] Awad K, Dalby M, Cree I, Challoner B, Ghosh S, Thurston D. The precision medicine approach to cancer therapy: Part 1 solid tumours. The Pharmaceutical Journal. 2019;**303**

[9] Barbour D. Precision medicine and the cursed dimensions. npj Digital Medicine. 2019;**2**. Article no. 4

[10] Martin W. High-Dimensional Statistics: A Non-Asymptotic Viewpoint. Cambridge, UK: Cambridge University Press; 2019

[11] Liu Q, Zhang N, Yang W, Wang S, Cui Z, Chen X, et al. A review of image recognition with deep convolutional neural network. In: Intelligent Computing Theories and Application. Proceedings of the 13th Intenrational Conference of Intelligent Computing. 2017. pp. 69-80

[12] Gutirrez L, Norambuena BK. A systematic literature review on word embeddings. In: Proceedings of the 7th International Conference on Software Process Improvement (CIMPS 2018). 2019. pp. 132-141

[13] Kussad Y, Kirkham D, Cassidy J, Patel N, Clifford H. Flatsomatic: A method for compression of somatic mutation profiles in cancer. 2019. Available from: https://arxiv.org/abs/1911.13259

[14] Kussad Y, Kirkham D, Cassidy J, Patel N, Clifford H. Learning embeddings from cancer mutation sets for classification tasks. 2019. Available from: https://arxiv.org/abs/1911.09008

[15] Bhlmann P, Kalisch M, Meier L. High-dimensional statistics with a view toward applications in biology. Annual Review of Statistics and Its Application. 2014;**1**:255-278

[16] Chalmers ZR, Connelly CF, Fabrizio D, Gay L, Ali SM, Ennis R, et al. Analysis of 100,000 human cancer genomes reveals the landscape of tumor mutational burden. Genome Medicine. 2017;**9**(1):34

[17] Omidiran D, Wainwright M. High-dimensional variable selection with sparse random projections: Measurement sparsity and statistical

efficiency. Journal of Machine Learning Research. 2010;**11**:2361-2386

[18] Cannings TI, Samworth RJ. Random-projection ensemble classification. Journal of the Royal Statistical Society, Series B: Statistical Methodology. 2017;**79**(4):959-1035

[19] Tibshirani R. Regression shrinkage selection via the lasso. Journal of the Royal Statistical Society, Series B. 2011; **73**:273-282

[20] Hanahan D, Weinberg R. The hallmarks of cancer. Cell. 2000;**100**: 57-70

[21] Brown A-L, Li M, Goncearenco A, Panchenko AR. Finding driver mutations in cancer: Elucidating the role of background mutational processes. PLoS Computational Biology. 2019; **15**(4):1-25

[22] Samstein R, Lee C-H, Shoushtari A, Hellmann M, Shen R, Janjigian Y, et al. Tumor mutational load predicts survival after immunotherapy across multiple cancer types. Nature Genetics. 2019;**51**:02

[23] Tajlic S, Litchfield K, Xu H. Insertion-and-deletion-derived tumour-specific neoantigens and the immunogenic phenotype: A pan-cancer analysis. The Lancet Oncology. July 2017;**18**:1009-1021

[24] Budczies J, Allguer M, Litchfield K, Rempel E, Christopoulos P, Kazdal D, et al. Optimizing panel-based tumor mutational burden (TMB) measurement. Annals of Oncology. 2019;**30**(9):1496-1506

[25] Bull K, Rimmer A, Siggs O, Miosge L, Roots C, Enders A, et al. Unlocking the bottleneck in forward genetics using whole-genome sequencing and identity by descent to isolate causative mutations. PLoS Genetics. 2013;**9**:e1003219

[26] Iengar P. Identifying pathways affected by cancer mutations. Genomics. 2017;**110**:12

[27] Chu D, Wei L. Nonsynonymous, synonymous and nonsense mutations in human cancer-related genes undergo stronger purifying selections than expectation. BMC Cancer. 2019;**19**:12

[28] Seagle B-L, Eng K, Yeh J, Dandapani M, Schultz E, Samuelson R, et al. Discovery of candidate tumor biomarkers for treatment with intraperitoneal chemotherapy for ovarian cancer. Scientific Reports. 2016; **6**:21591

[29] Zhang Y, Li H, Zhang W, Che Y, Bai W, Huang G. Lassobased coxph model identifies an 11lncrna signature for prognosis prediction in gastric cancer. Molecular Medicine Reports. 2018;**18**:10

[30] Guinney J, Wang T, Laajala TD. Prediction of overall survival for patients with metastatic castration-resistant prostate cancer: Development of a prognostic model through a crowdsourced challenge with open clinical trial data. The Lancet Oncology. 2017;**18**(1):132-142

[31] Benner A, Zucknick M, Hielscher T, Ittrich C, Mansmann U. High-dimensional cox models: The choice of penalty as part of the model building process. Biometrical Journal. 2010; **52**(1):50-69

[32] Witten DM, Tibshirani R. Covariance-regularized regression and classification for high dimensional problems. Journal of the Royal Statistical Society, Series B: Statistical Methodology. 2009;**71**(3):615-636

[33] Lin X, Huang X, Wang G, Tao W. Positive-definite sparse precision matrix estimation. Advances in Pure Mathematics. 2017;**07**:21-30

[34] Hu Z, Nie F, Tian L, Li X. A comprehensive survey for low rank regularization. Computing Research Repository. 2018. Available from: https://arxiv.org/abs/180804521

[35] Ye G, Tang M, Cai J-F, Nie Q, Xie X. Low-rank regularization for learning gene expression programs. PLoS One. 2013;**8**(12):1-9

[36] Yamada M, Takeuchi K, Iwata T, Shawe-Taylor J, Kaski S. Localized lasso for high-dimensional regression. In: Proceedings of the 20th International Conference on Artificial Intelligence and Statistics. Fort Laud-erdale, FL; 2017

[37] Diederik PK, Max W. Auto-encoding variational bayes. In: Proceedings of International Conference on Learning Representations. Scottsdale; 2013

[38] Zheng H, Yao J, Zhang Y, Tsang I, Wang J. Understanding vaes in fisher-shannon plane. In: Proceedings of the AAAI Conference on Artificial Intelligence. Vol. 33. 2019. pp. 5917-5924

[39] Way G, Greene C. Extracting a biologically relevant latent space from cancer transcriptomes with variational autoencoders. Pacific Symposium on Biocomputing. 2018;**23**:80-91

[40] Kompa B, Coker B. Learning a latent space of highly multidimensional cancer data. Pacific Symposium on Biocomputing. 2020;**25**:379-390

Chapter 4

Electronic Medical Records and Machine Learning in Approaches to Drug Development

Ayaka Shinozaki

Abstract

Electronic medical records (EMRs) were primarily introduced as a digital health tool in hospitals to improve patient care, but over the past decade, research works have implemented EMR data in clinical trials and omics studies to increase translational potential in drug development. EMRs could help discover phenotype-genotype associations, enhance clinical trial protocols, automate adverse drug event detection and prevention, and accelerate precision medicine research. Although feasible, data mining in EMRs still faces challenges. Existing machine learning tools may help overcome these bottlenecks in EMR mining to unlock new approaches in drug development. This chapter will explore the role of EMRs in drug development while evaluating the viability and bottlenecks of their uses in data mining. This will include discussions on EMR usage in drug development while highlighting successful outcomes in oncology and exploring ML tools to complement and enhance EMR as a widely accepted drug-research source, a section on current clinical applications of EMRs, and a conclusion to summarize and imagine what a future drug research pipeline from EMR to patient treatment may look like.

Keywords: drug research and development, machine learning, AI, electronic medical records, EMR, EHR, NLP, deep learning, big data, data analysis, data-mining

1. Introduction

Advances in Artificial Intelligence methods have skyrocketed in the past decade, especially in the medical space where the impact of healthcare reaches individuals across a broad spectrum of communities. In particular, machine learning (ML) researchers have gained access to a large quantity of high quality medical data, aggregated by health providers as a result of implementing hospital management systems. A crucial element of these management systems is electronic medical records (EMRs), which are rich in valuable real world data on patient, clinical and genomic data. An EMR is a digitized record of a medical occurrence documented either during or after an encounter by a medical professional in a medical environment. For example, the results of a blood test administered at a hospital may be part of an EMR. Clinical notes taken by the doctor in a routine check-up at a local clinic are also included in the EMR. EMRs can come in the form of structured data such as drug orders, medications, laboratory tests and diagnosis codes or unstructured data such as text-based clinical progress notes, radiology reports and pathology findings [1].

When EMRs are amalgamated to create a longitudinal overview of a specific patient, this larger unit of digitized records is called an electronic health record (EHR). Since EHRs contain historical data, they are used to track the health progression of patients over time. Although in some sources, the terms EMR and EHR are used interchangeably, or are sometimes referred to as the electronic patient record, for simplicity the above definitions are used here. Another digital record is the personal health record, which is the electronic medical data that the individual may choose to provide to the medical institutions or health providers, however issues of personal choice in volunteering data are beyond the scope of this chapter, so we do not consider the personal health record here.

Today, providers produce EMRs with the hope to provide a centralized source of medical data, which helps increase care coordination. With a standardized EMR system, if an individual decides to switch health providers, the medical data can seamlessly transfer to the new institutions. Furthermore, centralized medical data reduces duplication of records and identifies missing patient data, which reduces valuable time spent in clinical care. Compared to the traditional paperwork, EMRs significantly decreases disease identification time, making healthcare more time efficient and cost effective [2, 3]. In this sense, the EMRs improve quality of care.

In reality, there are issues in introducing EMRs into healthcare provider systems such as implementation and workflow disruptions. Implementation requires funding, necessary staff, and up to date digital technology. Institutions and geographic regions with ample resources will benefit from this implementation. However, for many smaller scale practices, implementation is not financially viable. For regions where institutions do not have access to technology that enables the production, storage and sharing of EMRs, this concept does not make sense. Furthermore, workflow is disrupted when clinicians and other medical professionals must alter their workflow in order to complete these documents. EMRs are notoriously unpopular in the medical community as it burdens professionals to constantly type on their computer instead of caring for their patients. Burdened professionals do not see the long term benefits and the reality in medical environments is that EMRs are primarily used for financial and administrative purposes. For example, although there are no global standards to what may be included in an EHR, it must always have billing codes, which are used for administrative purposes such as reimbursement or auditing reasons.

Despite these institutional challenges, EMRs are gaining traction in the biomedical space because there is potential to extract important biomedical conclusions from EMRs. As of December 2019, there are just under 2.1 million papers published on electronic medical records in drug development and research within google scholar [4]. Because EMRs are untapped and vast in quantity, researchers are particularly focused on testing ML methods on EMRs. EMRs also provide resources to carry out clinical trials at a lower cost and with reduced duration in terms of efficiency gained from automation and having better data sources. With a manual approach to identify and extract high value data, drug research on EMRs are not scalable and are extremely costly to employ domain experts for data extraction. The push for medical document digitization in conjunction with recent development in ML methods, such as natural language processing (NLP) that allows for machines to mimic human comprehension of written text, has allowed the outsourcing of these research tasks to machines and further facilitate drug research.

In the context of ML methods, EMRs pose problems such as how EMRs do not have a standardized formatting, how minorities could be underrepresented, and how EMRs contain human errors. Today in the healthcare space, EMRs exist in abundance but were not originally created with a large scale data-mining vision [5]. Rather, providers replaced paper-work with electronic records to keep up with the technological pace of the 21st century. Such digitization of the traditional paper-work was done on an ad-hoc basis and many healthcare institutions independently regulate EMRs to create a highly heterogeneous data set [6, 7]. This heterogeneity makes data pre-processing for ML methods time consuming and financially costly if domain experts are required for this task. Another difficulty stems from the issue of institutions and geographic regions not having access to technology or financial resources to implement EMRs. The lack of EMRs in particular communities means those individuals are not electronically visible. In this sense, EMRs will not be able to sample certain populations in the world. These underrepresented populations will not have as much benefit from the biomedical success of EMRs as those represented in the sample populations, increasing the inequality of medical care. Lastly, basic human error in the EMRs will affect analysis performed on these data sets, if they are not corrected. In addition, the EMRs come from different institutions, which may enter their data differently. Without a standardized requirement for EMRs, some parts will be missing core information and the operation is not scalable.

1.1 Chapter overview

This introduction started with a brief discussion of what an EMR is and how we define it in the absence of international unifying standards. This chapter will now move on to an overview of how machine learning techniques, applied to EMRs, are influencing three key areas of biomedical research and drug discovery: (1) phenotype-genotype associations, (2) clinical trials, and (3) pharmacovigilance.

Firstly, we assess the impact of EMRs on making accurate phenotype-genotype associations, where physical traits are linked to specific locus in the genome. We then look at EMRs in the context of clinical drug trials and pharmacovigilance, which together amount to the tracking of a drug's efficacy and adverse side-effects both before and after it is licensed and used. Finally, a number of different case studies are looked at in detail, and we present a vision of how integrated EMRs and ML-driven EMR drug research could be implemented in the future.

2. EMRs and phenotype-genotype association research

Phenotype-genotype association is the correspondence between a person's genetic makeup—their genotype, and the observable characteristics or pathologies that are a product of their genetics interacting with the environment—their phenotype. In the medical space, researchers study phenotype-genotype associations because variations in the human genome affect how a person exhibits phenotypic traits, so to understand phenotype-genotype relations is to have biological insight into disease mechanisms. Furthermore, phenotype-genotype associations are important in drug discovery because phenotype targets are used to identify viable drug targets within the human genome and are needed to understand the chemistry of a potential drug within the human biology. Understanding phenotype-genotype associations has useful downstream applications in many fields including disease categorization, phenotype discovery, pharmacogenomics, drug–drug interaction (DDI), and adverse drug event (ADE) detection, and genome-wide and phenome-wide association studies [8].

Phenotype-genotype association research owes its foundation to the genome-wide association studies (GWAS) studies that were driven by the potential of genetic variations modulating disease risks, expression and progression. Although the GWAS studies accumulated vast amount of genetic data, a remaining challenge is translating genetic markers to its associated phenotype [9, 10]. A high-throughput solution to such challenge is to harness phenotype data embedded in EMRs.

In a medical provider setting, clinical professionals observe phenotypes on a daily basis to diagnose diseases because phenotypic traits are manifestations of an individual's genome interacting with the environment. Such diagnosis is recorded extensively in EMRs, making them rich in phenotype-related data. Following the human genome project and the following development in sequencing whole genomes, EMRs can now feasibly link an individual's genome as part of their medical data.

However, linking genomic data to EHRs is not common in clinical practice. This is due to the combination of clinics offloading new sequencing technology to bioinformatics laboratories and the lack of infrastructure for integrating the processed genomic data into EHRs [11]. Unlike most clinical laboratory tests, genomic testing requires data curation during the bioinformatics pipelines. Therefore, when laboratories send genomic tests back to the original provider, the format or structure of that data may not be directly compatible with the local EHR system [12]. In 2016, laboratories were still physically mailing or faxing genomic reports in PDFs, which is a format that is extremely difficult for machines to read and interpret [12]. This clinical hurdle aside, in biomedical research this genomic inclusion in EHRs shows potential in secondary use as raw data from which to draw medically meaningful results [2, 12, 13]. Assuming that the EMR has adequate phenomic and genomic data on an individual, algorithms can translate raw data in EMRs to phenotype data, which in turn can be associated with the genomic data.

This section will focus on studies that cover phenotype-genotype research using EMRs that aims to advance drug research, with particular attention to the machine learning methods used in these cases. In a broad sense, this phenotype-genotype application of EMRs to drug research has two major tasks. First is to identify phenotypes contained in EMRs and second is to extract the phenotype to genotype associations.

One of the validated processes to identify phenotypic traits from EMRs is the use of standardized codes. Standardized codes have been designed for specific medical needs and are heavily used in the structured documentation in EMRs. When composing EMR's, medical professionals use an internationally standardized set of codes for reporting disease and health conditions called the International Classification of Disease (ICD) developed by the World Health Organization (WHO). For example, the ICD code may be a procedure code that indicates what medical procedures a patient has received during hospitalization or a disease code that specifies a clinician's diagnosis. Although standardized, the recorded ICD relies on a consistent interpretation of the ICD criteria for accuracy and relevancy, which will inevitably vary between clinicians, departments and institutions. However, researchers circumvent the larger issue of heterogenous EMR data types, which might range from character strings in clinical notes to matrices of pixels in radiology images, by focusing on these codes that are a standardized part of EHRs.

In the context of AI, using standardized codes is advantageous because they vastly reduce the set of possible inputs to any given machine learning algorithm. In practical terms, the data requires little pre-processing, since the codes already contain accurate and rich medical information described by domain experts. Computation becomes scalable as less pre-processing means less manual work involved, which is a necessity when extracting phenotypic data. Inevitably, there are a multitude of competing standards. As mentioned earlier, the ICD is consistently updated in order to internationally keep track of morbidity and mortality statistics with its eleventh version being adopted and replacing previous revisions starting 1 January 2022 [14]. In addition to the ICD, the US government has designed the ICD Clinical Modification (ICD-CM), which is based upon ICD but tailored to the US healthcare market. The Clinical Classification Software for ICD-CM, developed by the US Agency for Healthcare Research and Quality, is a further development to the ICD-CM that regroups codes into clinically relevant categories. New standards do not have to be based upon existing ones, however. Phecodes is a standard specifically designed for biomedical research and to facilitate phenome-wide association studies, first published in 2010 [15, 16]. In 2017, these different sets of standardized EMR codes (ICD, ICD-CM, phecodes) were compared based on their ability to create correctly pair single nucleotide polymorphism (SNP), which is a nucleotide level genetic variation, to the corresponding phenotype, and it was found that the phecodes performed markedly better than the ICD based standards [15, 17]. It is perhaps not surprising that the phecodes performed best. Phecodes were developed for research purposes, whereas ICD and related standards are more focused on record keeping and streamlining the financial aspect of healthcare. These results illustrate how common EMR codes used in hospitals are not well designed for ML purposes. Although these codes are a convenient aspect within the context of diverse data from EMRs, care must be taken when designing algorithms, which repurpose the codes for phenotype extraction.

EMRs often contain a mixture of standardized codes and free-text. To improve upon methods that only consider codes, machine learning tools, largely based upon NLPs, have been developed to collect more phenotypic data from data sources beyond standardized codes such as textual clinical notes, textual discharge summaries and radiology reports [1, 18–21]. Liao et al. developed a multimodal automated phenotyping (MAP) algorithm to leverage both ICD codes and EMR textual narratives based on the Unified Medical Language System [18]. MAP is multimodal because it can extract entities such as ICDs, medical NLP concepts and healthcare utilization information related to a certain phenotype from both codes and free text. Using MAP, Liao et al. analyzed those entities by different latent mixture models to predict whether a patient had a certain phenotypic feature. Liao et al. ran the algorithm through a validation dataset that contained labelled data with one of 16 unique phenotypes to show that MAP can extract relevant and phenotype-specific entities at comparable accuracy to those identified by a manual approach (AUC-MAP = 0.943, AUC-manual = 0.941). Another example of successful high throughput method to extract phenotypes from EMRs is PheNorm, which harnesses standardized codes as training labels and does not require domain experts to label the training set, making the model highly scalable and cost effective for phenotype research [19]. In the face of the ML hype, it is naive to say that ML methods are superior and domain experts will become superfluous in the future. For example, Coquet et al. demonstrated the use of NLP methods and a Convolutional Neural Network (CNN) method to create word embeddings in clinical notes to automate clinical phenotyping of prostate cancer patients [20]. In this particular case, the phenotyping accuracy of CNN model (F-measure = 0.918) surpassed that of the rule-based model (F-measure = 0.897) [20] and the authors concluded that the mixture of both models can lead to even better precision and accuracy. These statistics in which the CNN model, which is a class of deep neural networks, outperformed the rule-based model, an example of human driven modelling where domain knowledge is needed, is indicative of the potential in ML methods but human expertise is still needed to attain even higher accuracy and precision.

The next stage after phenotype extraction is to create phenotype-genotype associations. In addition to the development of higher quality and more available electronic medical records, EHRs can now be matched with biopsies stored in biobanks through patient-specific identifiers making it possible to study genetic and phenotypic data alongside clinical findings. Earlier studies focused on using statistical methods, such as the proof of concept study done by Denny et al. to develop a method to scan phenomic data for genetic associations using ICD billing codes [16]. Subsequent studies have shown the viability of using ML algorithms to understand phenotype-genotype associations using EMR sources with most of the papers published in the past year [22, 23]. Recently, deep learning gained popularity as an accurate framework at identifying phenotype-genotype associations [24]. Boudellioua et al. takes a deep neural network and developed an OpenSource phenotype-based tool called DeepPVP, which prioritizes potential causative variants from whole genome sequence data [25]. As another example, Zeng et al. used Bayesian network learning to extract epistatic interactions, which are gene-to-gene interactions that change exhibited phenotypic traits, that effect breast cancer patient survival on 1981 EHRs taken from the METABRIC dataset [26]. Their model learned SNP associations that effect breast cancer patient survival that agreed with domain knowledge from breast cancer oncologists [26]. Furthermore, unsupervised learning has also been recognized as a great tool to discover new phenotypes [27]. Stark et al. studied the unsupervised extraction of phenotypes from cancer clinical notes to use in association studies and reported success in finding new phenotype-genotype association hypothesis that are not published but plausible from a biological perspective [27]. Positive results form many recent studies demonstrates how deep learning shows promise in phenotype-genotype association extraction.

Such high performing machine learning on big data to create phenotype-genotype associations give hope to the future of personalized medicine, which is healthcare tailored to different variations in a genotypes. More basic biomedical research on phenotype-genotype associations opens possibilities for selecting best treatments and for studying drugs that come back with negative or adverse results. However, getting to such advanced levels of drug research is still on the horizon as there are still more challenges in finding phenotype-genotype associations.

As mentioned before, one of the major problems is that EMRs generally suffers from the difficulty in identification and correction of missing or mistaken data. In many cases, ML methods require large datasets and when EHRs are amalgamated from multiple sources, a high number of varying kinds of errors are carried over to the data set and therefore propagate through to the algorithms. Due to the high throughput of data in ML methods, there is a need for an automatic correction filter, or a complete work around the missing data. One solution to missing EMR data is to identify the missing phenotype data and correct it using a combination of bioinformatics and genomic data [28, 29]. Even with sparse numbers of high quality phenotypic or genotypic data, there has been studies that have successfully extracted phenotype-genotype information from EMR using semi-supervised, bulk phenotyping framework, and NLP-based machine learning techniques [24, 30, 31]. Another method to tackle missing data is to use a machine learning model to completely encompass the missing data as part of the training set and therefore accept the sparsity as part of the valid data [32]. Another solution is to acknowledge the missing data as a variable in the modelling of the algorithm and quantify its predicted effects on the final results and conclusion [33].

In summary, EMRs are a vital source of information in basic biomedical science, specifically for phenotype-genotype associations, and there is a trend to test ML methods on this untapped and vast data set to overcome the challenges EMRs face during data mining. The advantage of EMRs is that it can be mined for phenotypes and linked to genomic data. The section discussed different types of standardized codes used in EMRs, which are easy to pre-process for ML frameworks. Codes such as ICDs, ICD-CM, and phecodes showed that they can successfully and conveniently identify phenotypes. However, standard codes used by providers were not intended for data-mining purposes and therefore see performance issues when they are used outside their primary objective, to identify phenotypes. To harness EMR data beyond codes, studies look at a mixture of ICDs and free text. In the context of phenotype identification, this blend of data sources showed high performance especially when using ML methods in conjunction with more rule-based methods that require domain expertise. Furthermore, this section discussed the strong viability of ML methods for phenotype-genotype association identification, with a trend toward using deep learning frameworks. EMR applications through ML methods still face the problem of missing or erroneous data, which may affect the subsequent biomedical conclusions. Further work is being done to combat the shortcomings discussed and overall, EMRs have proven to be a promising data source for phenotype-genotype related research.

3. EMR use in clinical trials

Clinical research informatics has emerged in the last 5–6 years as a new field of biomedical translational research, which revolves around using informatics methods to collect, store, process and analyze real-world clinical data to further biomedical research purposes. With the increasing availability of such electronic data and the development of analysis tools, EMRs can help decrease the cost and time of clinical trials by automating patient recruitment, extend randomized control trials and enhance retrospective cohort studies.

Clinical trials are a crucial stage in drug development to test for drug safety and efficacy. These trials are time consuming, labor intensive and costly to operate, and a significant bottleneck for many trials is insufficient patient enrollment [34]. However, by harnessing the data contained within EMRs, clinical trials can become more efficient by automating recruitment and having a more extensive view of medical data compared to the traditional manual search. Successful examples have shown that EMR mining for potential recruitment are more cost efficient and less time consuming than traditional methods [35, 36]. As a quantitative example, a study done in the US studied 31 EHR-driven analysis on drug-to-genome interactions and concluded that EHRs helped decrease the trial cost by 72% per subject and reduced the duration of the studies [13].

It is also possible to repurpose systems that already exist within a clinical setting to improve trial recruitment. A study conducted by Devoe et al. repurposed an already existing Best Practice Alert (BPA) system, which was originally intended to improve patient care by automating basic keyword searches on patient EHRs, to recruit potential trial participants for a COPD study [37, 38]. Devoe et al. directly compared the cost effectiveness of the BPA-driven screening to that of the traditionally manual method, namely the EMR Reporting Workbench method where clinicians customize a query through a platform in order to pull data from the EHR database, and concluded that BPA was four times faster at screening all patients and ultimately lead to a projected 442.5 h reduction over the course of the study.

A particularly interesting case of a commercial EMR product developed for research purposes used in a clinical setting is a platform called InSite. This Software as a Service platform was developed out of the Electronic Health Record for Clinical Research (EHR4CR) project (completed Spring 2016), which aimed to create a secure, robust and scalable platform used around Europe to create a network of safe and security-compliant real world data, which can be reuse to further clinical research [39]. International research groups and medical providers from multiple countries developed this platform and intended for researchers to interact with hospital-based EHRs. A study by Claerhout et al. studied the feasibility of using InSite as a tool to estimate numbers of eligible participants for clinical trials at 24 European hospitals [40]. They studied the inclusion and exclusion (I/E) criteria of protocols from 23 trials across diverse therapeutic areas, including ABP 980 and trastuzumab for early breast cancer, a combination of cediranib and chemotherapy in relapsed ovarian, fallopian tube or epithelial cancer, and selumetinib in combination with docetaxel for metastatic lung cancer. These clinical trials were sponsored by various pharmaceutical companies [1] to represent key I/E criterion using terms included in the standard medical coding systems [2] [40]. It was found that a median of 55% of the I/E criteria can be translated to InSite queries using the standard medical coding systems to correctly identify potential trial patients. This result is promising as it shows the feasibility of translating the complex protocol criteria into machine-readable queries via an already existing platform.

This success of patient identification is attributed to how well defined the disease parameters are in the I/E criterion and whether its clinical concepts exactly match a query that the InSite platform can digest. Unfortunately, these queries do not contain easily accessible nor standardized temporal information on disease development such as the rapid progression of a tumor size or the timing at which an operation was carried out. This lack of temporal resolution led to the lowest formalization rate (38%) in patients with metastatic melanoma, revealing the difficulty of acquiring temporal information on tumor staging and genetic testing [40]. A possible next step to this study is to harness NLP to the unstructured EMR data and to resolve the temporal issue in order to increase performance in patient recruitment. Overall, this study showed the potential for this commercialized platform for optimizing recruitment by hospitals. Beyond the feasibility of estimating the number of potential trial patients, this platform is advantageous because InSite offers a convenient and efficient way for researchers can access real-time clinical data by extracting relevant EMRs without disrupting healthcare providers with new technological implementations.

It has been shown that NLP [34] is able to reduce the amount of manual-driven patient identification required. Once the number of patients eligible for a clinical trial is estimated, the next step is to carry out patient screening on each individual. There are three methods that can carry out these checks. Meystre et al. harnessed NLP to directly compare clinical trial screen accuracy between machine learning, rule-based and cosine-similarity based methods and reported the highest accuracy (micro-averaged recall 90.9%) and precision (89.7%) for the machine learning method [34]. In such automations, the usage of NLP and harnessing machine learning is key to fully automating cohort selections using EHRs, and there are research done to further those tools, which is illustrated with the emergence of CREATE [41] and SemEHR, which is an open source semantic search and analysis tool for EMRs [42]. Such automations revolutionize clinical trial processes by cutting down administrative work by an order of magnitude. To deal with the ever increasing amount of EMR data made available, case studies have also shown that unsupervised ML methods may be used to identify disease cohort selection with high accuracy compared to the traditional and manual methods [43].

In some cases, EMRs can allow for more diversity in clinical trials and provide data collection on individuals that are traditionally underrepresented, such as racial minorities, children, rural communities or pregnant women [35, 44, 45]. However,

---

1 Amgen, AstraZeneca, Bayer, Boehringer-Ingelheim, F-Hoffman La Roche, Janssen, Sanofi.

2 Diagnosis: ICD-10CM, procedures: ICD-PCS, medication: ATC, laboratory: LOINC, clinical findings: SNOMED and anatomic pathology/oncology ICD-O-3.

there are also studies that published poor performance of information retrieval through EMR and ML [46]. There are high expectations for a new wave of ML tools to revolutionize medicine but researchers must be vigilant for unexpected biases arising from ML models trained on skewed or bad data.

For an example of bias in EMR driven selection of patients for trial, we look at the work of Aroda et al. They compared EMR-driven recruitment for type 2 diabetes patient across multiple health centers in the US to that of the traditional manual method [47]. Although Aroda et al. reported that the EMR-based recruitment had higher numbers of patients screening, better performance and improved randomizations, they also noticed an association with fewer women and racial minorities recruited. EMR and electronic-driven recruitment may cause bias in the type of cohorts identified, as electronically visible individuals are more likely to be identified and then consent to trials. A skew in this electronic visibility allow only certain cohort groups to be identified and studied in a clinical trial [48].

These biases arising from ML models are a significant aspect of drug research as they may cause inadvertent negative effects when these technologies are brought to market and into the medical centers. This may be the case of poor data sets or a poor selection of algorithms. In the real world, catch-all algorithms that work in academia sometimes fail and sometimes there is just not enough data for the data-hungry machine learning methods. Since manual methods do not suffer due to lack of scale when ML-based and data-driven research fail when they cannot access big data, the rise of ML driven processes will not make manual ones totally obsolete.

Another potential for EMR is to extend short, cost-limited trials by electronically monitoring the cohort after the trial is over. This creates a long term follow up without the cost associated with a traditional, extended clinical trial. There has been a successful case in testing novel probiotics to carry out a 5 year follow up, which would have been too expensive in traditional methods and retention rate increased due to this electronic method [49]. Furthermore, EMR data may be used in clinical trials beyond just a follow-up. There is interest in using EMRs as a primary data source or as a feasibility assessment tool in observational clinical trials, comparative effectiveness studies and randomized clinical trials [50]. In addition, data can be used to carry out retrospective cohort studies or population based cohort studies. Kibbelaar et al. proposed a method to combine data from population-based registries with detailed EHR to conduct an observational study and reported on a case study in an hemato-oncology randomized registry trial [51].

These implementations are dependent on the patient's consent to partake in the trials and there are studies that investigate the process and ethics of such consent [52]. Beskow et al. identified patient informed consent as a bottleneck in using EHR for randomized clinical trials. A study has also identified gaps in ethical responsibility in clinical studies carried out [53]. Furthermore, compliance to security and privacy regulations is a critical challenge as clinically produced EMRs proliferate through cloud platforms, mobile devices and commercialized technology. Whilst security and data protection are of paramount importance when dealing with EMRs, a discussion of the methods currently in use is beyond the scope of this chapter. The reader is directed to Refs. [54–56], in which the current technologies and methods used for security measures on EMRs are reviewed.

To conclude, using data within EMRs can help decrease the cost and time of clinical trials. First, the section discussed successful examples of EMR mining for potential recruitment in clinical trials, which included using systems that already exist in clinical settings, such as BPA and InSite, and tools that employ ML methods. An advantage with the use of ML methods in clinical trials is the increase in diversity in trial patients but there is still an issue with the bias that cause inequality in patient selection. Ultimately, the quality of the ML approach depends on the quality of the training data. Therefore, with access to excellent data, EMRs can be used to extend short, financially limited trials or used as a primary data source to carry out aspects of data-driven clinical trials. Whilst ML methods are showing strong performance in enhancing clinical trials, big challenges remain before the data-driven method replaces the current clinical methodology.

4. EMR use in pharmacovalidation and data mining

However thoroughly a new drug is trialed and tested before it enters the market, it is possible that there are unknown adverse drug events (ADEs, colloquially known as side-effects) that manifest on time scales or in ways that cannot be seen in a clinical trial. Currently, adverse side effects of pharmaceutical products are a significant source for morbidity and are a significant healthcare cost in many countries [57, 58]. Therefore, it is vital that pharmaceutical companies undertake pharmacovigilance, in which they continually track the effects of their drugs after the drugs deployment. This means that clinical data on post-market drug effects has a high value to pharmaceutical companies [59]. Post-market surveillance of drugs to detect, evaluate and prevent ADEs with licensed drugs released in the market is called pharmacovigilance and is imperative for decreasing negative drug incidents.

Traditionally, medical professionals with domain knowledge would manually identify ADEs through sources such as clinical trials, health reports, published medical literature, observational literature and social media [60], which is time consuming and costly. Therefore, automatically mining these electronic narratives are an efficient way to identify negative events in the real world setting. Luckily, real world data on pharmaceutical products and their effects are richly logged in patient EHRs. To successfully mine the vast quantity of dense data in the EHRs for drug events, specifically ADEs, studies have focused on the narrative aspect of EMR and have successfully extracted ADE from both structured [61, 62] and unstructured [63–65] texts.

This focus on EHR narratives stems from studies that have shown that disease classification codes, such as ICD, used in EMRs do not encompass the symptoms, disease status and severity needed for ADE sensitivity and therefore are not appropriate in drug event mining [66–68]. Therefore it is necessary to extract more detailed information from the written text in EMRs, which is achieved using NLP algorithms. This is a two staged computational task. Firstly, the algorithm must perform accurate name entity recognition (NER) to identify diseases, drugs, and negative events in the text, and then it must quantify associations between those entities, to build a concept of what had occurred [69, 70].

Since 2012, significant developments in statistical analysis, machine-learning methods and heterogeneous data integration have allowed for automated ADE detection and offer tools for a novel, automated pharmacovigilance analytics [71]. Some statistical methods such as the odds ratio has been used by Leeper et al. and Banda et al. to create algorithms designed for extracting drug–ADE associations from EHRs [72, 73]. However, due to the need to define hypothesis using domain knowledge, experts in the field were necessary and this suggests a limitation that these statistical frameworks will not necessarily benefit from having more access to EHR resources because the core predictors depend on a priori knowledge, which is static within the algorithm. This means that there is currently still a manual element required in the process, which limits the scalability of this approach.

Some of the early EMR-narrative studies focused on keyword and phrase driven identification of general ADE. For example, there are semantic searches specializing in certain disease targets such as the work done by Ferrajolo et al. who looked at drug related acute liver injury [74, 75] and Pathak et al. who mined for DDI between cardiovascular and gastroenterology pharmaceutical products [76, 77]. Although these disease specific searches may increase ADE detection in a certain medical domain, this tailored approach is not scalable or translatable to other diseases. In terms of identifying general ADEs without a target disease, Honigman et al. developed a search method using the Micromedex M2 D2 (Micromedex, Denver, Colorado) medical data dictionary to semantically associate drugs and drug classes to their negative effects and successfully showed the viability of keyword searches on EMRs [78, 79]. Chazard et al. went a step further to demonstrate searches on a variety of data structures such as drug administration records, laboratory results, and other clinical records to successfully detect general ADEs within free texts [80, 81]. These previous methods successfully identified general ADEs, but keyword driven searches are now considered simplistic and not scalable, but the success of even that method shows that there is great promise for modern techniques.

A further development to keyword-based semantics is a more symbolic rule-based search that looks for semantic patterns around drug and ADE entities. These symbolic rule-based searches allow for more information on dosage and non-standard terminologies to be identified during queries and are more capable of general ADE recognition [82–85]. With the rise of semantic research in the medical space, biomedical NER and NLP has been developed to aid clinical semantic searches and there are several open sources available, which have been adapted for ADE identification such as MedLEE [86], MetaMap [87], cTAKES [88, 89], MedEx [90], and GATE [91]. Of those, MedLEE and MetaMap are two of the most widely used, particularly in the pharmacovigilance space, where researchers extract Unified Medical Language System (UMLS) concepts from texts using NLP based approaches. Studies have shown the adaptability of these already available NLP systems. Banerjee et al. used grammar rules to extract all noun entities and then used MetaMap to semantically identify the type of entity found. This study found that medications are easily found as entities, but the model had difficulty in extracting symptoms from laboratory test results as they vary in length and word choices [92]. In adapting these NLP systems, each study hit limitations of each source and in particular these tools are not very capable in temporal resolution, which makes it difficult to distinguish drugs that cause ADEs from those products that indicate the presence of an ADE.

This shortcoming in temporal resolution has pushed for another wave of studies. In understanding the use of medication and mentions of diseases, the context surrounding these entities will determine whether the drug was or was not used at a time before or after an adverse incident. Some studies have created time stamps on event entities and medication administration in order to exclude situations where the adverse symptom was an already existing condition at drug administration, the ADE was due to another drug, the drug did not cause the ADE and is mentioned as a negative association, or the pharmaceutical product was given as treatment to the ADE [84, 93, 94]. Although time resolution on ADE events increase the accuracy of adverse incident detection, the vagueness and implicit tendency in the human language to describe temporal events remain as bottlenecks [95].

A great example to illustrate a collaborative ML research on clinical EMRs is the MADE1.0 challenge carried out in the US. This ML challenge illuminated the popularity and effectiveness of deep neural networking learning in identifying negative drug incidents, as these models counted for most submissions to the competition.

4.1 MADE1.0 challenge: pharmacovigilance on cancer patient EMRs

In the US, death due to a drug incidence is one of the top six causes of death with around 2–5% of hospitalized patients suffering from ADEs; in each case an adverse event can increase healthcare cost by more than $3200 [96]. Traditionally, ADE-based pharmacovigilance is done by domain experts reading information on causality of drugs on incidents and temporal data on these events buried in the clinical narrative. However, this manual method is not scalable and very costly. To tackle the significant health and financial strain caused by ADEs, US research institutions participated in a machine learning challenge to develop methods automate real-time drug safety surveillance.

In 2018, University of Massachusetts (UMass) hosted a public NLP challenge to detect Medication and Adverse Drug Events from Electronic Health Records (MADE1.0). UMass provided 1092 longitudinal EHR notes, which were anonymized from 21 cancer patients from the University of Massachusetts Memorial Hospital. This EHR resource was rich with information on diseases, symptoms, indications, medications and relationships between these entities. Three main tasks were defined in this challenge: (1) named entity recognition (NER), which extracts drug medications, their attributes (dosage, drug administration, duration, etc.), disease indications, ADEs and severity, (2) relation identification (RI), which creates associations between entities, namely drug-indication, drug-ADE, and medication-attribute relations, and (3) the joint task that assess the NLP model's ability to perform both NER and RI. More detailed information on the challenge can be found at [96]. Jagannatha et al. reported that out of the 11 participating teams the highest F1 scores in each category was 0.8290 in NER, 0.8684 in RI, and 0.6170 in NER + RI, where the F1 score is the weighted mean of precision and recall with ranges from 0 (worst) up to 1 (best) [97].

Within NER task models, the main task can be distilled down to tokenizing sentences, so the tokens can then be labelled as specified entities. One common framework for NER is the hidden Markov model (HMM), in which the system is assumed to be the product of an unknown Markov process, which can then be statistically modelled. Conditional random fields (CRFs) are related to HMMs, however they differ in that, unlike HMMs, they are discriminative and classify labels by drawing decision boundaries. Unlike HMM, CRF does not have strict independence assumptions, which makes the model more flexible but highly complex at the training stage, meaning that retraining is more involved than that of the HMM [98]. The other main class of model is the neural network, including convolutional neural networks (CNN) and recurrent neural networks (RNN). Long short-term memory (LSTM) is an RNN architecture in common use for NER purposes. It is designed for classifications and predictions on time series data, in which events may occur with significant and unknown time lags in the sequence [99]. Teams involved in the MADE1.0 challenge used pre-trained embeddings to prepare the RNNs or as feature inputs into CRF training [97]. Within NER task models in this challenge, conditional random fields (CRF) and long short-term memory (LSTM) were among the most frequently used frameworks [97].

In the NER category, team WPI-Wunnava scored the highest scores with F1 = 0.8290 [97]. Wunnava et al. created a system called the Dual-Level Embeddings for Adverse Drug Event Detection (DLADE) to tailor to the NER task [100]. In the challenge, the NER task is limited to certain standard resources like NLTK, Stanford NLP, and cTakes for the text pre-processing for fairness of the participants with varying accessibility to resources. In particular, DLADE used training data and word embeddings provided by the challenge organizer as part of the publicly released resources. Wunnava et al. developed the system with a rule-based tokenizer, which first tokenized sentences, and then entities within sentences, where entities may be multiple words. The system then uses a combination of bi-LSTM, a model that examines the text sequence in the forward and reverse direction to extract contextual representation, for the initial two layers responsible for the character embedding and the word embedding but employed a linear-chain CRF for the output layer [100]. Wunnava et al. concluded that their dual-level character and word embedding method was a better approach compared to the simple word-embeddings by showing a statistically significant ($p < 0.05$ and $p < 0.01$) improvement in F1-score over multiple entities (ADE, drug, dose, duration, etc.) [100]. However, many challenges remain when identifying multi-worded entities, unknown abbreviations, ambiguous differentiation between entities such as indication vs. ADE, and uses of colloquial or non-medical jargon.

In both the RI and NER-RI tasks, the process can be simplified to a classification problem, where entity pairs are in a certain class of relationships. Research teams used a variety of approaches to the RI tasks. As well as neural network methods, they also used random forest classifiers, in which an ensemble of decision trees is used and the aggregate score from the committee of decision trees decides the output class. Support vector machines (SVM) were another popular tool; they are optimizing algorithms that maximize the margin between the support vectors (input data) and the decision hyperplane [101].

In the RI category, team UofUtah-Patterson score the highest scores with F1 = 0.8684 [97]. Chapman et al. treated the RI task as a two-step supervised classification problem and employed random forest models implemented on scikit-learn to identify true relations between entities and to class the type of relation of the identified pair [102]. Their source code for their models submitted to the MADE1.0 challenge can be found on their github page [103] and details on the model architecture is authored at [104].

In the NER + RI category, team IBMResearch-dandala obtained the highest integrated task score (F1 = 0.6170) by harnessing bidirectional long short-term memory (BiLSTM) and CRF neural network for medical entity recognition, and a combined BiLSTM and attention network for relation extraction [97]. Dandala et al. reported that NER was achieved at high accuracy (F = 0.83) and RI measured an F score of 0.87 achieved by adding joint modelling techniques and using external resources as extra data inputs [105]. However high the individual F score, the overall integrated task only reached 0.6170, which suggests the need for domain knowledge to increase accuracy in ADE detection.

The MADE1.0 challenge highlights the potential for developing pharmacovalidation based on ML methods with very high performance in categories such as NER and RI, which are crucial in automated ADE extraction from EMRs. At the time of completion of the MADE1.0 challenge, Jagannatha et al. suggested two broad approaches to further improve the challenge's outcomes [97]. First, to work on designing methods that include external knowledge and unlabeled text, which suggests the potential for unsupervised learning. The second point was to increase efforts in higher volume, labelled corpus to train the models on, but this does not solve the issue of algorithms failing to adapt to the messy, real world EHRs, an inevitable encounter in commercial use. Not only did this challenge show success in developing ML-based pharmacovigilance but also demonstrated the power of collaboration and influenced other groups to further ADE research.

4.2 Further ML works and trends on pharmacovigilance

After the MADE1.0 challenge, an even further increase of available EHR resources has pushed researchers to develop robust ML methods, which are inherently data hungry and are predisposed to the vast amount of information provided by clinical texts. There is a study that builds on the MADE1.0 challenge and shows the potential for deep learning models on EHR to extract ADE measures to help with pharmacovigilance. To try to solve the issue of under-reporting within the FDA Adverse Event Reporting System, Li et al. employed deep learning models and multi-task learning (MLT), in particular, hard parameter sharing, parameter regularization, and task relation learning, for ADE detection [106]. They used the MADE 1.0 challenge corpus, 1089 high-quality EMRs from oncology patients, for training and validation of their model. A BiLSTM conditional random field network was used for entity recognition and a BiLSTM-Attention network for entity relation extraction. Li et al. reported that the deep learning produced a F1 = 0.65 for the NER + RI task and this score was further improved through the hard parameter sharing MLT method to F1 = 0.67, whereas the other two MLTs did not improve performance. This study successfully built upon the findings from MADE1.0 and further improved the performance of the NER + RI task to show potential in this area.

Some ML trends that extract medically actionable results are the popularity of CRFs, SVMs, and random forest models. CRFs and SVMs may be used on languages beyond English. For example, Aramaki et al. studied Japanese clinical records and found that ADE were found in 7.7% of EHRs, out of which 59% can be automatically extracted [107]. They used CRFs and SVMs to determine whether a detected drug and adverse event pair was an ADE, which gave a 0.411 precision and 0.917 recall. In contrast, random forest models have been popular due to its reliable performance and explainability of the classifications when compared with other "black-box" models such as SVMs. Studies by Henriksson et al. and Wang et al. has used random forests for classification of entities and identify ADEs [108, 109]. Explainability of models is an often undervalued aspect of ML, but is valuable in the medical space. Overall, despite the many challenges, data-driven pharmacovigilance has advanced at an incredible pace owing to the mixture of funded challenges and developing ML methods and shows much promise to improve healthcare.

5. Drug repurposing

It is worth mentioning that EMR data can be mined for drug repurposing indications. The idea behind drug repurposing is to see whether existing, licensed drugs may have therapeutic benefits for conditions other than what they were designed for. Data-driven analysis is evidently key in this regard as it can detect drug response signals. Drug repurposing is different from the traditional drug discovery because data-driven analysis lacks a hypothesis for the indication intended to be treated or for the targeted biology. In other words, studies examine machine learning methods to see whether data-centric analysis can help create new hypothesis, which may either be a completely random and biologically impossible statement or a novel signal worthy of scientific investigation. Since drug repurposing only needs medical data and analytics, it is a cheap and quick alternative to the traditional drug discovery stages, which require basic research, pre-clinical research, clinical trials, and finally the review and approval of the pharmacogenomic product. The potential of drug repurposing is highly anticipated as this method requires big data and an increasing amount of digitized medical records such as EHRs are made available. It is a particularity popular topic in recent years as data-hungry machine learning tools develop and high-throughput server less machines are made cheaper and more accessible through cloud computing services such as AWS, Google Cloud Platform, and Microsoft Azure, to name a few. For a more in-depth discussion of oncology drug repurposing using data from EMRs, the reader is directed to Refs. [110–112].

6. Case studies in different countries

6.1 Oncology precision medicine in the US and Japan

Another anticipated but still young area is the possibility of precision medicine using individual genomic data. Cancer is an accumulation of genetic alternations within the cell and, oncogenetic or cancer-developing genes are called driver genes. Identifying driver genes within the genome and delivering the optimal treatment to such cancer-related targets is known as precision medicine. However, there is a vast amount of data within even a single individual's genome and finding variants becomes the key challenge in order to pinpoint the best pharmacological treatment for an individual based on their genetic background. Harnessing the combination of data from already existing genomic variant databases and historic clinical data from EMRs, researchers aim to find such cancer-related variations and driver genes. In a few countries, studies revolving around the interaction between the genome and cancer treatment drugs have gained much attention.

In the US, the NCI-MATCH trials, a phase II precision medicine cancer trial initiated in 2015, showed negative results in precision medicine and concluded that the genomic data did not correlate with any significant results in drug variation [113]. This low statistical significance is not surprising from a data mining perspective as numbers of patients accrued for each of the +40 arms within this study were very small, ranging from 4 to 70 people [114]. Furthermore, the majority of the recruited patients (62.5%) had rare tumors that were not the four most common cancers (breast, colorectal, non-small cell lung, and prostate) [115]. This diversity in cancer types may have introduced confounding factors that affected the statistics of the trial.

In Japan, starting 2018, the Japanese Ministry of Welfare and Labor is sponsoring a panel trial on partial genomic testing for oncogenetic variation. This partial genomic testing aims to reveal the best and optimal cancer drug treatment on the individual based on their genetic variations. In 2019, 11 Cancer Genomic Core hospitals and central medical institutions were selected to start collecting genomic data and clinical data in preparation for a nation-wide genomic panel trial [116]. Under the funding of the country's National Health Insurance, it strives to predict cancer patient treatment responses based on their partial genome data.

There is a complex interplay between intricate biological systems and the NCI-MATCH trial illustrates that precision medicine methods need much more development before they can pin point a certain genomic sequences to the onset of cancer. Some have voiced pessimistic views that this precision medicine task is not feasible and overly-costly at this point in time [117]. However, precision medicine is in the horizon. With more data samples, similar research can yield more insight into precision medicine.

In the future, individual whole genome data may be regular practice to include as part of EHRs in order to help deliver the optimal cancer treatment. Currently, there is a bottleneck where there are not enough types of commercialized cancer drug against which to test the genomic variation and to find which treatment works best on an individual. As all aspects of EMR-driven research converge, more medical data will be collected, stored and published. This will lead to already available commercial drugs undergoing more comprehensive pharmacovigilance and real-world data will effectively drive new drug research. Therefore, it is likely that more types of cancer pharmacology products will become available. Furthermore, the efforts in using ML to mine EMRs may lead to AI predicting cancer patient disease trajectories. The trend toward using NLP to extract relevant information from unstructured EMRs and harnessing deep learning could help reproduce drug-related clinical decision making carried out by medical professionals [110, 111].

6.2 Open sourced resources using EMRs in the UK

In England, there are trusts and clinical commissioning groups who oversee how providers such as hospitals and clinics use their resources. A problematic bottlenecks are that different trusts use different EMR platforms, which have little national standardization and do not allow for interprovider access, which especially cause problems when patients switch trust domains.

A remedy to this lack of standardization is the use of open sourced, publicly available resources including de-identified EMR data. Evident from the data-hungry nature of ML methods and their demonstrated need in scalable phenotype-genotype association research, publicly available EMRs play a crucial role in the advancement of this field. Some notable open sourced data sources and tools include the UK Biobank, where 50,000 individuals (aged 40–69) were recruited from England, Wales, Scotland [118]. The biobank includes detailed phenotype and genotype data, lifestyle surveys, pathophysiological data and imaging data on each individual [118]. Once a centralized, open-sourced EMR data is made available, the next step is the development of platforms that interact with said resource.

The CArdiovascular disease research using LInked Bespoke studies and Electronic health Records (CALIBRE) portal offers freely available software that provides tools and algorithms, which is research ready and have already extracted variables extracted from various EMRs. Phenotype algorithms contained in CALIBRE, which employs data from the UK Biobank, are rule based and use phenotype validations like etiological, which use external published evidence to support the algorithm; prognostic, which evaluate the event's similarity to already existing scientific knowledge; case-note review, which compares the positive predictive value (PPV) and the negative predictive value (NPV) against a gold standard like a clinician's notes; cross-EHR-source concordance, which checks the consistency in findings across other EHRs; genetic, which double checks whether there is consistency in genetic associations and external populations, which validates by comparing results to similar studies done in different countries [119]. These phenotype validations, and standardized validation systems in general, are crucial in characterizing ML algorithms since variations in training data can alter outputs even when the ML method does not change. As open source data proliferates, freely available validation methods may grow in a parallel manner.

In addition, openEHR is also a platform that pools industry specifications, clinical models and software that are intended for data science solutions in the healthcare space. OpenEHR was founded in 2003 by an international non-profit organization and maintained by individuals around the world [120]. In 2017, the UK became the first country to introduce infrastructure from openEHR into the main healthcare system to streamline phenotype data collection and vendor-neutral clinical data storage from all the trusts participating in the 100,000 genome project [121]. Newly coordinated pipelines of additional EHR data such as those from the NHS will increase the through-put in openEHR, which in turn develops the best tools to handle big data, which then completes the circle by promoting the use of an ever increasing amount of medical data. This data-driven vision, in which an open community encourages cooperation by open access and pools existing knowledge around EMR-driven healthcare, will certainly accelerate the evolution of ML methods.

6.3 EHR databases in Estonia

Estonia is one of the world-leading countries in terms of the nationwide systematization of digital medical documentation and the high quality of EHRs. By the end of 2014, Estonia had centralized EHR access via a single portal, where over 99% of the population could view their own medical records [122]. This is a remarkable statistic but more notably, Estonia's EHR vision had already been initiated in 2007 when the Estonian Genome Center of the University of Tartu established the foundations of the Estonian biobank, which includes 52,000 participants worth of genomic and health data representing about 5% of the adult population of Estonia [123, 124]. Seven years later, the Estonian biobank was linked to the Estonian National Health Information System (ENHIS), which included 44,000 inpatient and 212,000 outpatient medical summaries, EHRs and digital prescriptions from all medical service providers [124]. Since the merge, the databases have been updated through periodic additions of EHRs. By 2016, Estonia was ranked within the top three countries to have the best capability of effectively deploying, operating, maintaining and supporting statistical and medical research using EHRs by the HCQI Survey of Electronic Health Record System Development and Use [125]. This extensive data collection was made possible by the national electronic identification card (ID-card) as this chipped ID-card was made compulsory and became part of the national infrastructure [126]. As result of these efforts, Estonian EHR databases are highly valuable sources for researching EHR-driven methods.

An ADE study using Estonian EHR databases by Tasa et al. demonstrates the database's ability to conduct high impact, translational research. The whole-genome sequencing (WGS) data of +2200 Estonian Biobank participants and the EHRs of the sequenced individuals were taken from Health Insurance Fund Treatment Bills, Tartu University Hospital and North Estonia Medical Center databases [127]. EHRs were mined using ICD codes to find ADE occurrences and a mixture of the ICD and manual verification methods was used to identify associations between genetic polymorphisms and ADEs [127]. Associations between genetic variations and drug responses are vital in advancing personalized drug treatment, which is also referred to as pharmacogenomics. Important genes within the study of pharmacogenomics are called pharmacogenes. The study reported 29.1×10^6 novel variants. To priorities genetic analysis, Tasa et al. compiled 1314 loss-of-function, missense, and putative high-impact variants in promoter regions of 64 pharmacogenes [127]. They reported that 80.3% of the variants were rare (MAF $< 1\%$), and this high proportion suggests that gene variation is crucial in understanding pharmacogenomics [127]. Next, the study combined EHRs to the genetic data to extract 1187 participants with potential ADEs. As a validation, Tasa et al. replicated pharmacogenetic associations between the CYP2D6*6 allele and tramadol related ADEs ($p = 0.035$; odds ratio [OR] = 2.67) and between the same allele and amitriptyline induced ADEs ($p = 0.02$; OR = 6.0) [127]. In addition, they replicated four more validated pharmacogenetic associations and discovered nine independent, new gene associations with ADEs in a group of individuals divided by drug prescriptions. Notably, they identified a new association between CTNNA3 and myositis for oxicam-treated participants. This study demonstrated the viability of layering EHR and WGS data at a population-based scale in order to advance pharmacogenomic. Beyond the scope of this study, identifying pharmacogenomic associations relies more and more on big-data driven projects that looks for genetic variants in different communities and highlights variants that can be medically targeted to advance healthcare [128–130].

In summary, Estonia's world-leading efforts to integrate EHRs as a method to feedback data to basic research is a possible future of data-driven healthcare medicine, which focuses on digitization with a vision for translational biomedical research. Estonia created a data-mining driven database, in which different aspects of the EHRs are linked an ID-card. Although different implementations will be necessary to replicate Estonia's rich and accessible EHR database, Estonia sets a precedent to the rest of the world and demonstrates the positive biomedical implications of such well-organized databases of rich EHR sources.

7. Conclusion

In the past decade, EMRs have become a vital data source in advancing healthcare. In the context of AI, EMRs are highly attractive because there is a vast quantity of rich and variable data types which cannot be processed manually. In the context of biomedical research, EMRs have exciting potential for impactful medical applications, but only if actionable biomedical conclusions can be accurately extracted. In the clinical context, EMRs were introduced to replace the traditional paperwork but were not intended for data-mining research; they were never intended to perform anything that paper documents were not designed to do. Having been introduced in a time before the phrase "machine learning", digitization of medical records has far surpassed the imagined benefits of this transition. Envisioned as a direct replacement of paper records, EMR history has been fraught with difficulties: implementation costs, workflow disruptions and cyber-attacks to name a few. Harnessing EMRs for research purposes marks a milestone in translational biomedical medicine. It is the intersection of basic science, data-driven methods and clinical research where healthcare is transformed: every hospital visit improving human knowledge of diseases one EMR at a time.

The chapter started with a discussion of the EMRs definition, given that they have been introduced with little regard to compatibility with other existing EMR systems. There are many issues that hospitals can encounter when transitioning from paper records to electronic, however, efficiency gains from digitizing records are significant even without the use of big data. To exemplify what can be achieved by applying ML techniques to the data contained in EMRs, three key biomedical research areas were considered: phenotype-genotype association, clinical trials for new drug and pharmacovigilance studies.

Adopting high throughput data strategies into clinical drug trials can reduce the inefficiencies that often plague such trials. EMR mining using already existing systems can improve trial recruitment, but care must be taken to reduce potential bias in patient selection. Additionally, EMRs can be employed to continue data collection after the trial formally ends, a great benefit for financially limited trials, or they can even be treated as a primary data source as long as the data is considered to be of satisfactory standard.

After a drug undergoes clinical trials and is approved for market launch, pharmaceutical companies are encouraged to continue drug surveillance to detect, evaluate and prevent adverse drug events, which create medical and financial burdens. Such surveillance can be cheaply and efficiently done by continually mining EHR narratives. In the context of ADE detection, keyword searches are considered to be too simplistic and to lack scalability. Despite this, they still show some success in small scale studies, serving as a proof of concept that harnessing EHRs with more advanced processes could greatly benefit pharmagovigilance. However, NLP based-approaches performed much better than keyword-based methods and an excellent case study on NLP-driven pharmacovigilance is the MADE1.0 challenge. By bringing together multiple institutions, the challenge succeeded in developing high performing ML methods, including frequent usage of CRFs and LSTM, for the NER and RI tasks. This initiative promoted further works to create even more robust ML methods to extract ADEs from oncology EMRs and reflects the overall trend in the pharmacovigilance space toward CRF, SVM and random forest models.

With this vital context on how ML methods are used to analyze the data within EMRs, some selected international case studies on EHR-driven research were presented. Firstly, on the outlook of oncology precision medicine: NCI-MATCH trials in the US concluded that no drug response is correlated with genomic data, whilst preparation for partial genomic testing for oncology drugs is underway in Japan. Despite negative results nation-wide initiatives may spur on the collective development of drug research. Secondly, UK-based open source resources for EHR manipulation, were discussed, both large consolidated datasets and freely available tools, algorithms and platforms. This vision for open sourced resources is a valuable digital environment in which to pool technical knowledge, especially because of the translational and multi-disciplinary dimension of extracting medically meaningful conclusions from EHRs. Thirdly, the EHR databases set up in Estonia were reviewed, which are both nationally extensive and high quality. This set up the groundwork to deploy a population-based WGS and EHR combinatory study conducive to pharmacogenetic advances. Estonia's databases demonstrate the power of harnessing data from EHR for the progress of healthcare.

In contrast to the recent advancement and current interest in clinically-applied deep learning, there is still no definitive evidence of a model with predictive performance that is similar to a human physician [131]. As of 2020, there is no immediate vision in which AI can fully automate drug research pipelines or independently diagnose and provide subsequent health care procedures making researchers and clinicians obsolete. As we have seen, however, there is ample evidence that EMRs will increasingly play a vital role in all aspects of the drug research arc from fundamental science and clinical trials to post-market surveillance.

Conflict of interest

The author declares no conflict of interest.

Abbreviations

EMR	electronic medical record
EHR	electronic health record
NHS	National Health Services
ML	machine learning
DDI	drug–drug interaction
ADE	adverse drug event
ICD	International Classification of Disease
WHO	World Health Organization
ICD-CM	ICD Clinical Modification
SNP	single nucleotide polymorphism
CNN	convolutional neural network
I/E criteria	inclusion and exclusion criteria
NLP	natural language processing
HMM	hidden Markov model
CRF	conditional random fields
RNN	recurrent neural networks
LSTM	long short-term memory
BiLSTM	bidirectional long short-term memory
NER	named entity recognition

RI	relation identification
SVMs	support vector machines
CALIBRE	CArdiovascular disease research using LInked Bespoke studies and Electronic health Records
WGS	whole-genome sequencing

Author details

Ayaka Shinozaki[1,2,3]

1 techspert.io Ltd, Cambridge, UK

2 Department of Medicine, University of Cambridge, Cambridge, UK

3 Cancer Research UK, Cambridge Institute, Cambridge, UK

*Address all correspondence to: 13shinozakia@gmail.com

References

[1] Sharma H, Mao C, Zhang Y, Vatani H, Liang Y, Zhong Y, et al. Developing a portable natural language processing based phenotyping system. BMC Medical Informatics and Decision Making. 2019;**19**(3):78

[2] Bowton E, Field JR, Wang S, Schildcrout JS, Van Driest SL, Delaney JT, et al. Biobanks and electronic medical records: Enabling cost-effective research. Science Translational Medicine. 2014;**6**(234) 234cm3–234cm3. DOI: 10.1126/scitranslmed.3008604. Available from: https://stm.sciencemag.org/content/6/234/234cm3. ISSN: 1946-6234

[3] Kohane IS. Using electronic health records to drive discovery in disease genomics. Nature Reviews Genetics. 2011;**12**(6):417-428. DOI: 10.1038/nrg2999

[4] Google scholar. Available from: https://scholar.google.com/

[5] Evans RS. Electronic health records: Then, now, and in the future. Yearbook of Medical Informatics. 2016;**25**(S01): S48-S61

[6] Norton PT, Rodriguez HP, Shortell SM, Lewis VA. Organizational influences on health care system adoption and use of advanced health information technology capabilities. The American Journal of Managed Care. 2019;**25**(1):e21

[7] Sachdeva S, Bhalla S. Semantic interoperability in standardized electronic health record databases. Journal of Data and Information Quality (JDIQ). 2012;**3**(1):1-37

[8] Zeng Z, Yu D, Li X, Naumann T, Luo Y. Natural language processing for ehr-based computational phenotyping. IEEE/ACM Transactions on Computational Biology and Bioinformatics. 2018;**16**(1):139-153

[9] Marigorta UM, Rodríguez JA, Gibson G, Navarro A. Replicability and prediction: Lessons and challenges from gwas. Trends in Genetics. 2018;**34**(7): 504-517

[10] Allyn-Feuer A, Higgins GA, Athey BD. Pharmacogenomics in the age of gwas, omics atlases, and phewas. arXiv preprint. arXiv: 1808.09481, 2018

[11] Agarwala V, Khozin S, Singal G, O'Connell C, Kuk D, Li G, et al. Real-world evidence in support of precision medicine: Clinico-genomic cancer data as a case study. Health Affairs. 2018; **37**(5):765-772

[12] Warner JL, Jain SK, Levy MA. Integrating cancer genomic data into electronic health records. Genome Medicine. 2016;**8**(1):113

[13] Qian T, Zhu S, Hoshida Y. Use of big data in drug development for precision medicine: An update. Expert Review of Precision Medicine and Drug Development. 2019;**4**(3):189-200

[14] ICD-11 Implementation or Transition Guide. 2019. Available from: https://icd.who.int/docs/ICD-11ImplementationorTransitionGuide_v105.pdf

[15] Wei W-Q, Bastarache LA, Carroll RJ, Marlo JE, Osterman TJ, Gamazon ER, et al. Evaluating phecodes, clinical classification software, and ICD-9-cm codes for phenome-wide association studies in the electronic health record. PLoS ONE. 2017;**12**(7):1-16. DOI: 10.1371/journal.pone.0175508

[16] Denny JC, Ritchie MD, Basford MA, Pulley JM, Bastarache L, Brown-Gentry

K, et al. PheWAS: Demonstrating the feasibility of a phenome-wide scan to discover gene–disease associations. Bioinformatics. 2010;**26**(9):1205-1210. ISSN: 1367-4803. DOI: 10.1093/bioinformatics/btq126

[17] Hebbring SJ, Rastegar-Mojarad M, Ye Z, Mayer J, Jacobson C, Lin S. Application of clinical text data for phenome-wide association studies (PheWASs). Bioinformatics. 2015; **31**(12):1981-1987. ISSN: 1367-4803. DOI: 10.1093/bioinformatics/btv076

[18] Liao KP, Sun J, Cai TA, Link N, Hong C, Huang J, et al. High-throughput multimodal automated phenotyping (map) with application to phewas. bioRxiv. 2019. DOI: 10.1101/587436

[19] Yu S, Ma Y, Gronsbell J, Cai T, Ananthakrishnan AN, Gainer VS, et al. Enabling phenotypic big data with phenorm. Journal of the American Medical Informatics Association. 2017; **25**(1):54-60

[20] Coquet J, Bozkurt S, Kan KM, Ferrari MK, Blayney DW, Brooks JD, et al. Comparison of orthogonal NLP methods for clinical phenotyping and assessment of bone scan utilization among prostate cancer patients. Journal of Biomedical Informatics. 2019;**94**: 103184

[21] Zeng Z, Espino S, Roy A, Li X, Khan SA, Clare SE, et al. Using natural language processing and machine learning to identify breast cancer local recurrence. BMC Bioinformatics. 2018; **19**(17):498

[22] Pikoula M, Quint JK, Nissen F, Hemingway H, Smeeth L, Denaxas S. Identifying clinically important COPD sub-types using data-driven approaches in primary care population based electronic health records. BMC Medical Informatics and Decision Making. 2019; **19**(1):86

[23] Zhou S-M, Fernandez-Gutierrez F, Kennedy J, Cooksey R, Atkinson M, Denaxas S, et al. Defining disease phenotypes in primary care electronic health records by a machine learning approach: A case study in identifying rheumatoid arthritis. PLoS ONE. 2016; **11**(5):e0154515

[24] Zeng Z, Deng Y, Li X, Naumann T, Luo Y. Natural language processing for EHR-based computational phenotyping. IEEE/ACM Transactions on Computational Biology and Bioinformatics. 2019. ISSN: 2374-0043; **16**(1):139-153. DOI: 10.1109/TCBB.2018.2849968

[25] Boudellioua I, Kulmanov M, Schofield PN, Gkoutos GV, Hoehndorf R. DeepPVP: Phenotype-based prioritization of causative variants using deep learning. BMC Bioinformatics. 2019;**20**(1):65

[26] Zeng Z, Jiang X, Neapolitan R. Discovering causal interactions using bayesian network scoring and information gain. BMC Bioinformatics. 2016;**17**(1):221

[27] Stark SG, Hyland SL, Fernandes Pradier M, Lehmann K, Wicki A, Perez Cruz F, et al. Unsupervised extraction of phenotypes from cancer clinical notes for association studies. arXiv preprint. arXiv:1904.12973, 2019

[28] Salcedo CC, Labilloy G, Andrew S, Hwa V, Tyzinski L, Grimberg A, et al. OR07–6 integrating targeted bioinformatic searches of the electronic health records and genomic testing identifies a molecular diagnosis in three patients with undiagnosed short stature. Journal of the Endocrine Society. 2019;**3** (Suppl 1). ISSN: 2472-1972. DOI: 10.1210/js.2019-OR07-6

[29] Tong J, Huang J, Chubak J, Wang X, Moore JH, Hubbard RA, et al. An augmented estimation procedure for EHR-based association studies

accounting for differential misclassification. Journal of the American Medical Informatics Association. 2020;**27**(2):244-253. ISSN: 1527-974X. DOI: 10.1093/jamia/ocz180. ocz180

[30] Beaulieu-Jones BK, Greene CS. Semi-supervised learning of the electronic health record for phenotype stratification. Journal of Biomedical Informatics. 2016;**64**:168-178. ISSN: 1532-0464. DOI: 10.1016/j.jbi.2016.10.007

[31] Chiu P-H, Hripcsak G. EHR-based phenotyping: Bulk learning and evaluation. Journal of Biomedical Informatics. 2017;**70**:35-51. ISSN: 1532-0464. DOI: 10.1016/j.jbi.2017.04.009

[32] Hubbard RA, Huang J, Harton J, Oganisian A, Choi G, Utidjian L, et al. A bayesian latent class approach for EHR-based phenotyping. Statistics in Medicine. 2019;**38**(1):74-87. DOI: 10.1002/sim.7953

[33] Beesley LJ, Fritsche LG, Mukherjee B. A modeling framework for exploring sampling and observation process biases in genome and phenome-wide association studies using electronic health records. bioRxiv. 2018. DOI: 10.1101/499392. Available from: https://www.biorxiv.org/content/early/2018/12/20/499392

[34] Meystre S'e M, Heider PM, Kim Y, Aruch DB, Britten CD. Automatic trial eligibility surveillance based on unstructured clinical data. International Journal of Medical Informatics. 2019; **129**:13-19

[35] Hurdle JF, Haroldsen SC, Hammer A, Spigle C, Fraser AM, Mineau GP, et al. Identifying clinical/translational research cohorts: Ascertainment via querying an integrated multi-source database. Journal of the American Medical Informatics Association. 2012;**20**(1):164-171

[36] Obeid JS, Beskow LM, Rape M, Gouripeddi R, Black RA, Cimino JJ, et al. A survey of practices for the use of electronic health records to support research recruitment. Journal of Clinical and Translational Science. 2017;**1**(4): 246-252

[37] Devoe C, Gabbidon H, Schussler N, Cortese L, Caplan E, Gorman C, et al. Use of electronic health records to develop and implement a silent best practice alert notification system for patient recruitment in clinical research: Quality improvement initiative. JMIR Medical Informatics. 2019;**7**(2):e10020

[38] Bejjanki H, Mramba LK, Beal SG, Radhakrishnan N, Bishnoi R, Shah C, et al. The role of a best practice alert in the electronic medical record in reducing repetitive lab tests. ClinicoEconomics and Outcomes Research: CEOR. 2018;**10**:611

[39] Electronic health records for clinical research (ehr4cr). Available from: http://www.ehr4cr.eu/

[40] Claerhout B, Kalra D, Mueller C, Singh G, Ammour N, Meloni L, et al. Federated electronic health records research technology to support clinical trial protocol optimization: Evidence from ehr4cr and the insite platform. Journal of Biomedical Informatics. 2019; **90**:103090

[41] Liu S, Wang Y, Wen A, Wang L, Hong N, Shen F, et al. Create: Cohort retrieval enhanced by analysis of text from electronic health records using omop common data model. arXiv preprint. arXiv:1901.07601, 2019

[42] CogStack. Cogstack/cogstack-semehr. Available from: https://github.com/CogStack/SemEHR

[43] Glicksberg BS, Miotto R, Johnson KW, Shameer K, Li L, Chen R, et al. Automated disease cohort selection using word embeddings from electronic

health records. In: Pacific Symposium on Biocomputing; World Scientific. 2018. pp. 145-156

[44] Horowitz CR, Sabin T, Ramos M, Richardson LD, Hauser D, Robinson M, et al. Successful recruitment and retention of diverse participants in a genomics clinical trial: A good invitation to a great party. Genetics in Medicine. 2019;**21**: 2364-2370

[45] Devers K, Gray B, Ramos C, Shah A, Blavin F, Waidmann T. The Feasibility of Using Electronic Health Records (EHRs) and Other Electronic Health Data for Research on Small Populations. Urban Institute: Washington; 2013

[46] Chamberlin SR, Bedrick SD, Cohen AM, Wang Y, Wen A, Liu S, et al. Evaluation of patient-level retrieval from electronic health record data for a cohort discovery task. MedRxiv. 2019;**1**:19005280

[47] Aroda VR, Sheehan PR, Vickery EM, Staten MA, LeBlanc ES, Phillips LS, et al. Establishing an electronic health record–supported approach for outreach to and recruitment of persons at high risk of type 2 diabetes in clinical trials: The vitamin D and type 2 diabetes (d2d) study experience. Clinical Trials. 2019; **16**(3):306-315

[48] Pfaff E, Lee A, Bradford R, Pae J, Potter C, Blue P, et al. Recruiting for a pragmatic trial using the electronic health record and patient portal: Successes and lessons learned. Journal of the American Medical Informatics Association. 2018;**26**(1):44-49

[49] Davies G, Jordan S, Brooks CJ, Thayer D, Storey M, Morgan G, et al. Long term extension of a randomised controlled trial of probiotics using electronic health records. Scientific Reports. 2018;**8**(1):7668

[50] Cowie MR, Blomster JI, Curtis LH, Duclaux S, Ford I, Fritz F, et al. Electronic health records to facilitate clinical research. Clinical Research in Cardiology. 2017;**106**(1):1-9

[51] Kibbelaar RE, Oortgiesen BE, Van Der Wal-Oost AM, Boslooper K, Coebergh JW, Veeger NJGM, et al. Bridging the gap between the randomised clinical trial world and the real world by combination of population-based registry and electronic health record data: A case study in haemato-oncology. European Journal of Cancer. 2017;**86**:178-185

[52] Beskow LM, Brelsford KM, Hammack CM. Patient perspectives on use of electronic health records for research recruitment. BMC Medical Research Methodology. 2019;**19**(1):42

[53] Goldstein CE, Weijer C, Brehaut JC, Fergusson DA, Grimshaw JM, Horn AR, et al. Ethical issues in pragmatic randomized controlled trials: A review of the recent literature identifies gaps in ethical argumentation. BMC Medical Ethics. 2018;**19**(1):14

[54] McDermott DS, Kamerer JL, Birk AT. Electronic health records: A literature review of cyber threats and security measures. International Journal of Cyber Research and Education (IJCRE). 2019;**1**(2):42-49

[55] Ganiga R, Pai RM, Pai MMM, Sinha RK. Security framework for cloud based electronic health record (EHR) system. International Journal of Electrical & Computer Engineering. 2020;**10**:2088-8708

[56] Farhadi M, Haddad H, Shahriar H. Compliance checking of open source EHR applications for HIPAA and ONC security and privacy requirements. In: 2019 IEEE 43rd Annual Computer Software and Applications Conference (COMPSAC), Vol. 1; IEEE. 2019. pp. 704-713

[57] Onder G, Pedone C, Landi F, Cesari M, Vedova CD, Bernabei R, et al.

Adverse drug reactions as cause of hospital admissions: Results from the Italian group of pharmacoepidemiology in the elderly (GIFA). Journal of the American Geriatrics Society. 2002; **50**(12):1962-1968. DOI: 10.1046/j.1532-5415.2002.50607.x

[58] Salas-Vega S, Haimann A, Mossialos E. Big data and health care: Challenges and opportunities for coordinated policy development in the eu. Health Systems & Reform. 2015; **1**(4):285-300

[59] Mehta N, Pandit A. Concurrence of big data analytics and healthcare: A systematic review. International Journal of Medical Informatics. 2018;**114**:57-65

[60] Harpaz R, Callahan A, Tamang Y, Low S, Odgers D, Finlayson S, et al. Text mining for adverse drug events: The promise, challenges, and state of the art. Drug Safety. 2014. ISSN: 1179-1942; **37**(10):777-790. DOI: 10.1007/s40264-014-0218-z

[61] Cami A, Arnold A, Manzi S, Reis B. Predicting adverse drug events using pharmacological network models. Science Translational Medicine. 2011. ISSN: 1946-6234;**3**(114) 114ra127–114ra127. DOI: 10.1126/scitranslmed.3002774. Available from: https://stm.sciencemag.org/content/3/114/114ra127

[62] Pouliot Y, Chiang AP, Butte AJ. Predicting adverse drug reactions using publicly available pubchem bioassay data. Clinical Pharmacology & Therapeutics. 2011;**90**(1):90-99. DOI: 10.1038/clpt.2011.81

[63] Liu M, Wu Y, Chen Y, Sun J, Zhao Z, Chen X-w, et al. Large-scale prediction of adverse drug reactions using chemical, biological, and phenotypic properties of drugs. Journal of the American Medical Informatics Association. 2012;**19**(e1): e28-e35

[64] Zheng H, Wang H, Xu H, Wu Y, Zhao Z, Azuaje F. Linking biochemical pathways and networks to adverse drug reactions. IEEE Transactions on Nanobioscience. June 2014. ISSN: 1558-2639;**13**(2):131-137. DOI: 10.1109/TNB.2014.2319158

[65] Harpaz R, Vilar S, DuMouchel W, Salmasian H, Haerian K, Shah NH, et al. Combing signals from spontaneous reports and electronic health records for detection of adverse drug reactions. Journal of the American Medical Informatics Association. 2012;**20**(3): 413-419

[66] Nadkarni PM. Drug safety surveillance using de-identified EMR and claims data: Issues and challenges. Journal of the American Medical Informatics Association. 2010. ISSN: 1527-974X (Electronic); 1067–5027 (Print); 1067–5027 (Linking);**17**(6): 671-674. DOI: 10.1136/jamia.2010.008607

[67] Classen DC, Resar R, Griffin F, Federico F, Frankel T, Kimmel N, et al. 'Global trigger tool' shows that adverse events in hospitals may be ten times greater than previously measured. Health Affairs. 2011;**30**(4):581-589. DOI: 10.1377/hlthaff.2011.0190

[68] Doupi P. Using EHR data for monitoring and promoting patient safety: Reviewing the evidence on trigger tools. Studies in Health Technology and Informatics. 2012;**180**: 786-790

[69] Luo Y, Riedlinger G, Szolovits P. Text mining in cancer gene and pathway prioritization. Cancer Informatics. 2014;**13**(Suppl 1):69-79

[70] Cohen KB, Demner-Fushman D. Biomedical Natural Language Processing. Amsterdam, The Netherlands: John Benjamins; 2014. Available from: https://www.jbe-platform.com/content/books/9789027271068

[71] Luo Y, Thompson WK, Herr TM, Zeng Z, Berendsen MA, Jonnalagadda SR, et al. Natural language processing for EHR-based pharmacovigilance: A structured review. Drug Safety. 2017;**40**(11): 1075-1089. ISSN: 1179-1942. DOI: 10.1007/s40264-017-0558-6

[72] Leeper NJ, Bauer-Mehren A, Iyer SV, LePendu P, Olson C, Shah NH. Practice-based evidence: profiling the safety of cilostazol by text-mining of clinical notes. PLoS ONE. 2013;**8**(5): e63499

[73] Banda JM, Callahan A, Winnenburg R, Strasberg HR, Cami A, Reis BY, et al. Feasibility of prioritizing drug–drug-event associations found in electronic health records. Drug Safety. 2016;**39**(1):45-57

[74] Ferrajolo C, Verhamme KMC, Trifirò G, Jong G W't, Giaquinto C, Picelli G, et al. Idiopathic acute liver injury in paediatric outpatients: Incidence and signal detection in two European countries. Drug Safety. 2013; **36**(10):1007-1016

[75] Ferrajolo C, Coloma PM, Verhamme KMC, Schuemie MJ, de Bie S, Gini R, et al. Signal detection of potentially drug-induced acute liver injury in children using a multi-country healthcare database network. Drug Safety. 2014;**37**(2):99-108

[76] Pathak J, Kiefer RC, Chute CG. Using linked data for mining drug-drug interactions in electronic health records. Studies in Health Technology and Informatics. 2013;**192**:682

[77] Pathak J, Kiefer RC, Chute CG. Mining drug-drug interaction patterns from linked data: A case study for warfarin, clopidogrel, and simvastatin. In: 2013 IEEE International Conference on Bioinformatics and Biomedicine; IEEE. 2013. pp. 23-30

[78] Honigman B, Lee J, Rothschild J, Light P, Pulling RM, Yu T, et al. Using computerized data to identify adverse drug events in outpatients. Journal of the American Medical Informatics Association. 2001;**8**(3):254-266

[79] Honigman B, Light P, Pulling RM, Bates DW. A computerized method for identifying incidents associated with adverse drug events in outpatients. International Journal of Medical Informatics. 2001. ISSN: 1386-5056; **61**(1):21-32. DOI: 10.1016/S1386-5056(00)00131-3. Available from: http://www.sciencedirect.com/science/article/pii/S1386505600001313

[80] Chazard E, Băceanu A, Ferret L, Ficheur G. The ADE scorecards: A tool for adverse drug event detection in electronic health records. Studies in Health Technology and Informatics. 2011;**166**:169-179

[81] Chazard E, Ficheur G, Bernonville S, Luyckx M, Beuscart R. Data mining to generate adverse drug events detection rules. IEEE Transactions on Information Technology in Biomedicine. 2011;**15**(6): 823-830

[82] Epstein RH, Jacques PS, Stockin M, Rothman B, Ehrenfeld JM, Denny JC. Automated identification of drug and food allergies entered using non-standard terminology. Journal of the American Medical Informatics Association. 2013;**20**(5):962-968

[83] Eriksson R, Jensen PB, Frankild S, Jensen LJ, Brunak S. Dictionary construction and identification of possible adverse drug events in Danish clinical narrative text. Journal of the American Medical Informatics Association. 2013;**20**(5):947-953

[84] Eriksson R, Werge T, Jensen LJ, Brunak S. Dose-specific adverse drug reaction identification in electronic patient records: Temporal data mining

in an inpatient psychiatric population. Drug Safety. 2014;**37**(4):237-247

[85] Roitmann E, Eriksson R, Brunak S. Patient stratification and identification of adverse event correlations in the space of 1190 drug related adverse events. Frontiers in Physiology. 2014;**5**:332

[86] Friedman C, Shagina L, Lussier Y, Hripcsak G. Automated encoding of clinical documents based on natural language processing. Journal of the American Medical Informatics Association. 2004;**11**(5):392-402

[87] Aronson AR. Effective mapping of biomedical text to the umls metathesaurus: The metamap program. In: Proceedings of the AMIA Symposium. American Medical Informatics Association. 2001. p. 17

[88] Savova GK, Masanz JJ, Ogren PV, Zheng J, Sohn S, Kipper-Schuler KC, et al. Mayo clinical text analysis and knowledge extraction system (ctakes): Architecture, component evaluation and applications. Journal of the American Medical Informatics Association. 2010; **17**(5):507-513

[89] Re'ategui R, Ratt'e S. Comparison of metamap and ctakes for entity extraction in clinical notes. BMC Medical Informatics and Decision Making. 2018;**18**(3):74

[90] Xu H, Stenner SP, Doan S, Johnson KB, Waitman LR, Denny JC. Medex: A medication information extraction system for clinical narratives. Journal of the American Medical Informatics Association. 2010;**17**(1): 19-24

[91] Cunningham H. Gate, a general architecture for text engineering. Computers and the Humanities. 2002; **36**(2):223-254

[92] Ritwik B, Ramakrishnan IV, Henry M, Perciavalle M. Patient centered identification, attribution, and ranking of adverse drug events. In: 2015 International Conference on Healthcare Informatics. IEEE. 2015. pp. 18-27

[93] Liu Y, LePendu P, Iyer S, Shah NH. Using temporal patterns in medical records to discern adverse drug events from indications. AMIA Summits on Translational Science Proceedings. 2012; **47**:2012

[94] LePendu P, Iyer SV, Bauer-Mehren A, Harpaz R, Mortensen JM, Podchiyska T, et al. Pharmacovigilance using clinical notes. Clinical Pharmacology & Therapeutics. 2013;**93**(6):547-555

[95] Sun W, Rumshisky A, Uzuner O. Temporal reasoning over clinical text: The state of the art. Journal of the American Medical Informatics Association. 2013;**20**(5):814-819

[96] Umass bionlp projects. Available from: https://bio-nlp.org/index.php/projects/39-nlpchallenges

[97] Jagannatha A, Liu F, Liu W, Yu H. Overview of the first natural language processing challenge for extracting medication, indication, and adverse drug events from electronic health record notes (made 1.0). Drug Safety. 2019;**42**(1):99-111

[98] Sutton C, McCallum A, et al. An introduction to conditional random fields. Foundations and Trends® in Machine Learning. 2012;**4**(4):267-373

[99] Olah C. Understanding LSTM networks. Available from: https://colah.github.io/posts/2015-08-Understanding-LSTMs/

[100] Wunnava S, Qin X, Kakar T, Rundensteiner EA, Kong X. Bidirectional LSTM-CRF for adverse drug event tagging in electronic health records. In: International Workshop on Medication and Adverse Drug Event Detection. 2018. pp. 48-56

[101] Berwick R. An idiot's guide to support vector machines (SVMS). Available from: http://web.mit.edu/6.034/wwwbob/

[102] Chapman AB, Peterson KS, Alba PR, DuVall SL, Patterson OV. Detecting adverse drug events with rapidly trained classification models. Drug Safety. 2019;**42**(1):147-156

[103] Burgersmoke. burgersmoke/made-crf. 2019

[104] Chapman AB, Peterson KS, Alba PR, DuVall SL, Patterson OV. Hybrid system for adverse drug event detection. In: International Workshop on Medication and Adverse Drug Event Detection. 2018. pp. 16-24

[105] Dandala B, Joopudi V, Devarakonda M. Adverse drug events detection in clinical notes by jointly modeling entities and relations using neural networks. Drug Safety. 2019; **42**(1):135-146

[106] Li F, Liu W, Hong Y. Extraction of information related to adverse drug events from electronic health record notes: Design of an end-to-end model based on deep learning. JMIR Medical Informatics. 2018;**6**(4):e12159

[107] Aramaki E, Miura Y, Tonoike M, Ohkuma T, Masuichi H, Waki K, et al. Extraction of adverse drug effects from clinical records. Medinfo. 2010;**160**: 739-743

[108] Henriksson A, Zhao J, Boström H, Dalianis H. Modeling electronic health records in ensembles of semantic spaces for adverse drug event detection. In: 2015 IEEE International Conference on Bioinformatics and Biomedicine (BIBM); IEEE. 2015. pp. 343-350

[109] Wang G, Jung K, Winnenburg R, Shah NH. A method for systematic discovery of adverse drug events from clinical notes. Journal of the American Medical Informatics Association. 2015; **22**(6):1196-1204

[110] Srivastava S, Soman S, Rai A, Srivastava PK. Deep learning for health informatics: Recent trends and future directions. In: 2017 International Conference on Advances in Computing, Communications and Informatics (ICACCI); IEEE. 2017. pp. 1665-1670

[111] Wu Y, Warner JL, Wang L, Jiang M, Xu J, Chen Q, et al. Discovery of noncancer drug effects on survival in electronic health records of patients with cancer: A new paradigm for drug repurposing. JCO Clinical Cancer Informatics. 2019;**3**:1-9

[112] Chang Y, Park H, Yang H-J, Lee S, Lee K-Y, Kim TS, et al. Cancer drug response profile scan (CDRscan): A deep learning model that predicts drug effectiveness from cancer genomic signature. Scientific Reports. 2018;**8**(1): 8857

[113] Nci-match precision medicine clinical trial. Available from: https://www.cancer.gov/about-cancer/treatment/clinical-trials/nci-supported/nci-match

[114] Nci-match/eay131-ecog-acrin. 2020. Available from: https://ecog-acrin.org/trials/nci-match-eay131

[115] Nci-match trial releases new findings. Available from: https://www.cancer.gov/news-events/press-releases/2018/nci-match-first-results

[116] Oncoguide NCC oncopanel system insurance developed by the national cancer center. Available from: https://www.ncc.go.jp/jp/information/pr_release/2019/0529/index.html

[117] OF PRECISION. The Precision-Oncology Illusion. 2016

[118] Uk biobank. Available from: https://www.ukbiobank.ac.uk/

[119] Denaxas S, Parkinson H, Fitzpatrick N, Sudlow C, Hemingway H. Analyzing the heterogeneity of rule-based EHR phenotyping algorithms in caliber and the Uk biobank. BioRxiv. 2019:685156

[120] Open industry specifications, models and software for e-health

[121] Heard S, Beale T. Available from: https://www.openehr.org/openehr_in_use/deployed_solutions_detail/27

[122] Gheorghiu B, Hagens S. Use and maturity of electronic patient portals. Studies in Health Technology and Informatics. 2017:136-141

[123] Leitsalu L, Haller T, Esko T, Tammesoo M-L, Alavere H, Snieder H, et al. Cohort profile: Estonian biobank of the Estonian Genome Center, University of Tartu. International Journal of Epidemiology. 2014;**44**(4): 1137-1147

[124] Leitsalu L, Alavere H, Tammesoo M-L, Leego E, Metspalu A. Linking a population biobank with national health registries—The estonian experience. Journal of Personalized Medicine. 2015; 5(2):96-106

[125] Oderkirk J. Readiness of Electronic Health Record Systems to Contribute to National Health Information and Research. 2017

[126] Sepper R, Ross P, Tiik M. Nationwide health data management system: A novel approach for integrating biomarker measurements with comprehensive health records in large populations studies. Journal of Proteome Research. 2010;**10**(1):97-100

[127] Tasa T, Krebs K, Kals M, Mägi R, Lauschke VM, Haller T, et al. Genetic variation in the estonian population: Pharmacogenomics study of adverse drug effects using electronic health records. European Journal of Human Genetics. 2019;**27**(3):442

[128] Esplin ED, Oei L, Snyder MP. Personalized sequencing and the future of medicine: Discovery, diagnosis and defeat of disease. Pharmacogenomics. 2014;**15**(14):1771-1790

[129] Relling MV, Evans WE. Pharmacogenomics in the clinic. Nature. 2015;**526**(7573):343

[130] Ramos E, Doumatey A, Elkahloun AG, Shriner D, Huang H, Chen G, et al. Pharmacogenomics, ancestry and clinical decision making for global populations. The Pharmacogenomics Journal. 2014; **14**(3):217

[131] Chen D, Liu S, Kingsbury P, Sohn S, Storlie CB, Habermann EB, et al. Deep learning and alternative learning strategies for retrospective real-world clinical data. NPJ Digital Medicine. 2019;**2**(1):1-5

Section 3

Drug Repurposing and Clinical Trials

Chapter 5

Applications of Machine Learning in Drug Discovery II: Biomarker Discovery, Patient Stratification and Pharmacoeconomics

John W. Cassidy

Abstract

Cancer remains a leading cause of morbidity and mortality around the world. Despite significant advances in our understanding of the pathology of the disease, and the substantial public and private investment into treatment development, late-stage patients often exhaust therapeutic options. Indeed, in the US alone, there were >1.7 million new cancer diagnoses and >600,000 cancer-associated deaths in 2019. As biology in general and cancer research in particular become ever richer in data, we explore the role of machine learning (ML) in changing the cancer drug development landscape. In the first part of this analysis, we focussed on ML for target identification and drug design. We discussed the growing need for ML-based analysis as we enter an age of clinical -omic data and provided a primer to ML-based techniques for the non-statistician/mathematician. In this chapter, we will explore the problem of tumour heterogeneity together with the role of ML in the discovery and development of cancer biomarkers and for clinical trial design. We end with a brief consideration of the economics of personalised cancer treatment.

Keywords: machine learning, biomarker discovery, oncology

1. Introduction

The cancer therapeutic market was estimated to reach $98.9 billion USD in 2018, with a compounded annual growth rate of 7.7%. The cost of individual cancer drugs is similarly rising at a rate well above inflation. Ipilimumab, for example, was priced at $120,000 on launch, despite providing an overall survival benefit of just 4 months. More generally, if we correct for inflation and increased survival benefit, the average cost of new cancer therapies increased at $8500 per year from 1995 to 2013 [1]. If we continue along this path of yearly incremental price increases in new therapies approved, while not seeing associated health benefits, public opinion may begin to further question the moral standing of the pharmaceuticals industry [2].

However, there exists a profound conflict at the heart of the pharmaceutical industry. The efficiency of the drug development process is falling, leading to higher costs to be recovered per approved drug. At the same time, research into the biological underpinnings of disease are making it clear that pathologies once

IntechOpen

thought of as a single disease are incredibly heterogeneous in nature [3]. In such cases, personalised medicine may be the best method for treating diseases like cancer, which could shrink the available markets for each individual drug.

Cancer has been known to be heterogeneous since experimental pathologists began to study tumour in detail at the turn of the nineteenth century. First, differences in cellular morphology were described [4], followed by surface marker expression [5] and later growth rates [6] and response to therapy [7]. Recently, high throughput profiling of DNA, RNA and protein expression in human cancers has helped uncover the true scale of this diversity [8]. For example, early work in breast cancer enabled stratification of patients based on the presence of oestrogen receptor alpha (ERα), which led to the successful targeting of tamoxifen for ERα-positive (ERα+) patients [9]. More recent work has enabled comprehensive stratification of breast and other cancers [8, 10]. In breast cancer, a 50-gene signature (PAM50) can now be used to stratify patients into four intrinsic subtypes (luminal A, luminal B, HER2-enriched and basal-like) with distinct clinical outcomes [11, 12]. Taking this stratification effort further, researchers at the University of Cambridge integrated copy number (CN) data with transcriptomics to uncover 11 distinct Integrative Clusters of breast cancer [10].

Patient stratification improves the taxonomy of cancer, which is the initial step towards better understanding of the drivers of tumour growth and consequently towards improved precision medicines [13]. However, as our appreciation of stratification and heterogeneity increases, the challenge for pharmaceutical companies is to develop an economic model that enables them to provide personalised treatment to patients at a sustainable cost.

In practice, the efficiency of the drug development process has been dropping for a number of years. The average time for taking a new therapeutic to market is often stated as 10 years; however, in reality this often ranges from 3 to 20 years [14]. If we consider the average cost of developing a new drug, in 2014 the Tufts Center for the Study of Drug Development estimated this at $2.6 billion [14]. A large proportion of this cost is associated with a 90% attrition rate in Phase I–Phase III trials; $2.6 billion covers the nine failures for every one approved drug. However, on an individual pharmaceutical company basis, the picture can get even worse. AstraZeneca has recently spent an average of $11 billion per registered drug [15]. Considering (1) high upfront costs, (2) high risk of overspending and failure and (3) the possibility of very long development time frames, pharmaceutical companies must price in the cost of capital to their calculation of drug price. $11bn spent over 20 years, when that money could have been generating 10% annual returns in a stock market index, means that it is not uncommon for pharmaceutical companies to wish to generate many tens of billions of dollars in lifetime drug sales.

Thankfully, we are entering a world of big data biology and techniques like machine learning (ML) can help us increase efficiency in the drug discovery and development process. In the first part of our analysis, *Applications of Machine Learning in Drug Discover I: Target Discovery and Small Molecule Drug Design*, we discussed how molecular target identification and small molecule lead optimisation can be improved though computational techniques. However, early development accounts for a relatively small proportion of the total costs associated with drug development. Phase III trials alone, for example, on average cost over $100 million [16]. If we are to improve efficacy in drug development, we must improve late-stage clinical trials and stratification of patients post market approval.

In this chapter, we discuss how ML is allowing high personalisation of treatment strategies.

First, we consider the causes of tumour heterogeneity, its genomic underpinnings and the latest research into patient stratification. Next, we consider the discovery of predictive biomarkers for patient stratification in clinical trials and post market approval. Thankfully, the same techniques we use to improve trials can also be used to fulfil precision oncology and deliver better patient outcome. As the number of drugs increases, we may also be able to use repurposing and repositioning to make up for lost revenues from personalisation and increase profitability of old drugs. Lastly, we discuss computational pathology as one of the most obvious early uses of ML in cancer diagnosis. We end with a forward-looking discussion of the future of precision oncology and what this means for the pharmaceutical industry.

2. The causes and consequences of tumour heterogeneity

Cancer is a disease of the genome [13, 17]. Through the normal course of ageing, cells acquire somatic mutations as a consequence of intrinsic processes or the exposure to exogenous mutagens. These changes in the cellular DNA can directly influence the structure and function of transcribed proteins, and, in some cases, confer a survival advantage ('fitness'), on the cell. Peter Nowell postulated in 1976 that heterogeneous fitness in a niche could lead to Darwinian competition and selection among clones [18], and that successive clonal expansion was the origin of a tumour. This theory was supported by early evidence that genetic aberrations were the cause of a tumour's phenotypic traits [19] and more recent genomics research [8, 20].

It is now accepted that tumours harbour various layers of genomic complexity and the resultant heterogeneity can have profound effects on disease progression. Moreover, genomic instability, which fuels the diversity essential for any Darwinian process is intertwined with both the development and maintenance of tumour heterogeneity, and the clinical consequences thereof [21, 22]. Indeed, both inter- and intratumour heterogeneity can be explained by the genomic instability inherent to a tumour's biology and the sequential acquisition of driver mutations. Though changes in a tumour's microenvironment (e.g. increase in inflammation or immune cell infiltrate) or epigenetic regulation (e.g. MLH1 promotor methylation in microsatellite unstable CRC) are undoubtedly required to transform a clonal expansion of benign cells into a malignancy [17, 23].

Interestingly, a series of studies over the last couple of years from the Sanger Institute have shed new light onto the clonal origins of human cancers. First, in 2013, it was shown by Alexandrov and colleagues that distinct mutational processes (e.g. exposure to tobacco smoke and exposure to ultraviolet light) led to distinct mutational signatures in human cancer [24]. Next, Martincorena and colleagues showed that outwardly normal human skin not only had traces of these mutational signatures but in some cases harboured daughter cells of past clonal expansion events [25]. This was later corroborated in other tissues including the oesophagus [26]. It was not until 2020, when a study by Colom et al. [27] was published that we had any insight into what differentiated these clonal populations from bona fide premalignant clones. In an elegant study, the authors showed that when an expanding mutant clone occupied the same niche as one of similar 'fitness', each clone's proliferative advantage decreases, and the niche reverts towards balanced proliferation and differentiation that characterises normal tissue homeostasis [27]. Such studies highlight how far we have come in our understanding of the causes of tumour heterogeneity since Peter Nowell's seminal work in 1976 [18], and how much we may still have to learn.

Tumour heterogeneity has a very real clinical consequence: chemotherapy and targeted agents do not have uniform efficacy. This holds across malignancies of different subtype and even between cells of the same tumour [28]. As mentioned, for example, breast cancers can be clinically stratified based on heterogeneity in the presence of hormone receptors (ERα/PR) and HER2, the presence of which define treatment recommendation.

As the cost of DNA sequencing and other high throughput profiling technologies continues to drop, our taxonomy of cancer is becoming ever more nuanced [29]. Early genomic classifications based on single parameters have evolved into complex integrative methodologies designed to capture heterogeneity across multiple levels, such as the 11 Integrative Clusters of breast cancer defined by Curtis et al. [10]. Indeed, as multi-parameter stratification improves, we are beginning to stratify both breast [30] and colorectal cancers [31] based on immune infiltrates and immunogenomic signatures. Such classification will have a direct influence on our use of novel immunotherapies [32].

A second clinical consequence of tumour heterogeneity is in the development of resistance to targeted therapies [33]. Typically, this results from the outgrowth of specific pre-existing populations within a tumour rather than from *de novo* evolution [3, 34]. It therefore stands to reason that the higher the more pronounced the clonal heterogeneity in a tumour, the wider the pool from which drug-resistant clones may evolve [3]. There exists a fine balance within a tumour between waves of clonal expansion by hyper-fit cells, and the maintenance of subclones from which resistance can develop. Such an association between tumour heterogeneity and drug resistance has been noted in ovarian [35] and oesophageal [21] cancers.

Evolution occurs when spatial or temporal selective pressure is applied to populations with differential fitness, which is itself underwritten by heritable features. Drug treatment induces evolution of clonal populations within a tumour, which can provide a niche into which resistant clones can grow. Counterintuitively, however, anti-cancer therapies do not necessarily lead to a reduction in overall clonal diversity or tumour genomic heterogeneity [36]. For example, in a study of 47 breast cancer patients, strong changes in cellular phenotype were seen before and after chemotherapy, with no corresponding changes in genetic diversity, implying that a shift in the epigenomic landscape had resulted from exposure to chemotherapeutic selective pressures [37]. In addition, several studies have identified the role of transient epigenetic states in the resistance to cancer therapy. For example, Sharma et al. consistently detected a subpopulation of cells with >100-fold reduced erlotinib sensitivity across a panel of eight cancer cell lines [38]. The authors found that this drug-tolerant phenotype was transiently acquired and lost by individual cells within the population in a process linked to IGF-1 signalling and histone demethylase-mediated chromatin remodelling [38].

Genomic instability is the driving force of tumour heterogeneity. Although intratumour heterogeneity is linked with poor patient outcome, genomic instability is only associated with poor prognosis to a point. A recent study examined 1000 treatment-naïve tumours and found that the total number of genomic clones had significant association with overall survival [39]. However, the authors note that high clone number was only indicative of survival up to a maximum clonal diversity of four. Indeed, a diversity of more than four subclones was associated with longer overall survival [39, 40]. The authors used a 10% cell frequency cut off in their studies, yet, they are rare clonal populations which are thought to have evolved most recently [41] and may be more associated with resistance to targeted therapy [42–44]. This could go some way to explaining the apparent discrepancy seen between this, and other studies.

Hence, both intra- and intertumour heterogeneity have profound clinical consequences in terms of differential response to therapy, development of drug resistance and disease progression. Beyond stratified medicine, a better understanding of the causes and consequences of clonal heterogeneity within a tumour will allow a deeper understanding of the emergence of drug resistance. New analysis tools such as the REVOLVER package could empower researchers to stratify patient groups based on the basis of how their tumour evolved [45, 46] and perhaps allow prediction of a tumour's evolutionary trajectory and a corresponding therapeutic strategy. Moreover, a greater understanding of genomic instability and its contribution to treatment resistance, and sensitivity, is needed.

3. Predictive biomarkers for personalised cancer care

As discussed, late-stage clinical trials are one of the most expensive, in terms of resource spending and time, in the total drug development lifecycle. Although many predictive models are mentioned in the literature, few have been validated in clinical trials. Various limitations around model performance, validation and dataset availability are currently limiting translation [47].

As one of the key clinical endpoints, drug sensitivity or efficacy would be one of the most important metrics to predict from preclinical data in order to improve the clinical success rate of drugs. In terms of real-world evidence, a handful of groups have now published case studies where biomarkers derived from ML-driven predictive modelling have played a central role in the discovery and development of new therapeutic agents [48–50].

In one such case study, Li and colleagues built drug sensitivity models from cancer cell lines treated with erlotinib [an EGFR protein kinase inhibitor approved for NSCLC patients with activating mutations: exon 19 deletion (del19) or exon 21 (L858R) substitution] and sorafenib (a non-specific kinase inhibitor approved for advanced renal cell carcinoma) [48, 51]. Models were then used to stratify patients in the BATTLE (Biomarker-integrated Approaches of Targeted Therapy for Lung Cancer Elimination) clinical trial [48, 52], with identified biomarkers backwards justified with knowledge of the mechanism of action of each kinase inhibitor drug. Crucially, combining biomarker-driven adaptive trials such as BATTLE with basket trials (tissue of origin agnostic), we can move towards truly data-driven personalised oncology. Indeed, the FDA approved pembrolizumab [a programmed cell death 1 (PD1) inhibitor] in 2017 for tumours of a specific genetic background rather than site of origin [53]. This is the first instance of a cross-indication approval based solely on a genetic biomarker and highlights the need for further study in drug repurposing and data-driven biomarker discovery for the future of genomic cancer medicine.

To address some barriers to model translation into clinical practice, several community efforts have been attempted to help evaluate and standardise ML-based models. For example, the FDA launched a validation initiative for benchmarking ML models for predicting clinical endpoint from RNA expression data [54]. In this Microarray Quality Control II (MAQC II) initiative, teams were tasked with generating predictive models for several clinical endpoints in a multiple myeloma dataset. The most effective method used a univariant Cox regression model to identify a gene signature associated with individuals at high risk of low overall survival [55]. Though the authors note that arbitrary cut offs in overall survival may have limited effectiveness (24 months was the cut off for high risk, despite overall survival being a continuous variable suited to Cox modelling). A similar approach can be taken with breast cancer gene expression data to predict overall survival as a continuous variable [46]. Interestingly, the multiple myeloma prognostic biomarker developed was later independently validated by several groups [56–58].

The NCI-DREAM challenge was a similar community-driven effort to provide standardised datasets for benchmarking ML models [59]. In this case, models were trained on a dataset consisting of RNA expression profiles, mutation data (from SNP array), protein array data, exome sequencing and DNA methylation, from 35 breast cancer cell lines treated with 31 anti-cancer drugs. The models then had to predict outcome from a blinded dataset of 18 cell lines with the same 31 drugs. The best performing models were invariably regression based: such as the kernel method, nonlinear regression, regression trees, sparse linear regression, partial least squares regression, principal component regression and ensemble methods [59]. The dataset continues to be used to benchmark a variety of models such a random forest ensemble frameworks [60], group factor analyses [61] and other approaches [62, 63].

Our group has approached the problem of data availability by combining datasets from multiple sources (DNA, RNA; patients, cell lines) using variational autoencoders (VAE) optimised to compress somatic mutations while maintaining signal [64]. We trained our models on somatic profiles from 8062 Pan-Cancer patients from The Cancer Genome Atlas and 989 cell lines from the COSMIC cell line project and compared two different neural network architectures for the VAE: multilayer perceptron (MLP) and bidirectional LSTM. We found that the size of the latent space did not have a significant effect on the VAE learning ability and showed that the model maintained representations of 64 dimensions and held the same predictive power as the original 8298-dimension vector, through prediction of drug response [64].

Stratification of cancer patients into molecular subgroups in an effort to predict drug sensitivity is a common practice. As discussed previously, one such method integrated copy number, gene expression and mutational data from >2000 breast cancers in order to define 11 'Integrative Subtypes' [10]. In a later study from the same authors, a biobank of breast cancer xenografts (PDX models) was established and high throughput combinatorial drug screens were performed on xenograft-derived tumour cells [65, 66]. The authors observed differential sensitivity between PDX models of different integrative clusters and even observed drugs with similar molecular mechanisms of action to cluster together [67]. However, in general the reproducibility and clinical relevance of unsupervised clustering is poor. This is thought to be attributable to the routine analysis of small cohorts consisting of fewer than 100 patients, together with the use of biased traditional consensus clustering techniques. In our study, we combined multiple RNA expression datasets and developed a robust Monte-Carlo Consensus Clustering program, called PDACNet. We identified six biologically novel subtypes that were reproducible across datasets [67].

ML-based predictive biomarkers have also seen recent advances outside of the oncology space. Leveraging the rich UK biobank dataset, for example, Paré and colleagues were able to explain 46.9% of overall polygenetic variance for height and 32.7% for body mass index (BMI) through the building of gradient boosted regression trees based on SNP arrays [68]. Expanding this beyond SNP arrays, Khera and colleagues built ML-driven polygenic risk score to identify individuals with greater than threefold increased risk for coronary artery disease (80% of the population were found to be genetically predisposed), atrial fibrillation (6.1%), type 2 diabetes (3.5%), inflammatory bowel disease (3.2%) and breast cancer (2.5%) [69].

Building from polygenic risk scores to multi-omic profiling, Tasaki and colleagues studied clinical remission in rheumatoid arthritis patients by longitudinal monitoring of the drug response at multi-omics levels in the peripheral blood of patients [70]. This high dimensional phenotyping, coupled with ML-led analysis, enabled the authors to uncover signatures independently associated with resistance to treatment and with no known associated with previously discovered disease severity indexes. This technique could be expanded to a quantitative measure of molecular remission useful in a clinical setting.

Perhaps among the most exciting use of ML in driving our understanding of human pathophysiology is in the building of *in silico* experimental models in which researchers may perturb regulatory networks at will and illicit real (but simulated) biological responses. Towards this goal, Way and Greene built a VAE model trained on over 10,000 tumours across 33 different cancer types from The Cancer Genome Atlas (TCGA) named 'Tybalt' [71]. The authors showed Tybalt could capture biologically relevant features and model cancer gene expression under perturbation. Though a lot of future work is needed, such system-based approaches could 1 day aid in prediction of specific activated expression patterns that resulted from genetic changes or perturbation by therapeutics. Combined with discussed survival and outcome-based predictive models, we could then model treatment response to myriad theoretical combination therapies *in silico*.

Though the discussed examples of ML-led biomarker discovery are promising, there are several key barriers to adoption that still require work. End clinical users, for example, cite interpretability of the classifier as a critical barrier for clinical adoption. We must also validate our models in the context of multi-site, multi-institutional datasets to demonstrate their generalisability.

4. Adaptive clinical trials

As stated, the most capital and time-intensive part of brining a new medicine to market is arguably the late-stage clinical trial. Phase III studies, for example, can run over multiple years and across multiple clinical centres and cost upwards of $100 million. As advanced statistical techniques gain traction, and as our understanding of biomarkers of response improves, we could see dramatic overhaul in the way clinical trials are carried out.

One set of designs of particular interest to this chapter are the adaptive clinical trials. Adaptive designs utilise results accumulating through the course of a trial to modify the trial's course in accordance with pre-specified rules. Pre-specified changes to the trial design may include refining the sample size, abandoning treatments or doses, changing the ratio of patients in each arm (e.g. placebo arm), focussing recruitment efforts in patients most likely to benefit or stopping the entire trial early either successfully or due to a lack of efficacy [72]. In this way, adaptive trials can be more capital and time efficient, more informative and more ethically acceptable than those of a traditional fixed design.

As adaptive trials could theoretically rely on sequential decision-making, they could be particularly well suited to ML-based efficiency gains. Indeed, there is a class of algorithms inspired by clinical trials themselves, known as Multi-Arm Bandit (MAB) algorithms [73]. MABs are useful when a fixed and limited set of resources must be allocated between alternative (competing) choices in a way that maximises total reward, even though the reward for each choice is not immediately known to the MAB. Thus, MABs can find a set of choices to maximise reward with incomplete information through reinforcement learning. Given the fixed nature of a classical clinical trial, in which groups patients are given treatments sequentially one after another, MAB algorithms could be natural candidates to help guide further phases of drug testing [47, 74].

As the simplest form of a MAB system, we can consider a Phase III clinical study to comprise K treatment arms, each with an unknown probability of success ($p1, p2, \ldots pK$) and a reward (Xt) equal to 1 if treatment succeeds and 0 if treatment fails. The choice of treatment for the tth patient depends on each of the previously given treatments and their observed outcomes. The trial's data-driven adaptivity could therefore allow statistical power for each arm to be reached with fewer patients by incorporating automatic interim analysis in the treatment decision. Theoretically, such a trial would be resource efficient across all parameters (time, economic, minimise side effects, maximise patient life) [74].

Despite the theoretical promise of adaptive trials, clinical uptake has been slow. This could be due to statistical requirements for traditional trials, for example balancing prognostic covariates in each arm [74], or could be due to practical difficulties such as the significant delay in feedback on treatment effectiveness [75]. It is for this reason that we can look forward to the maturation of technologies such as the real-time monitoring of treatment effectiveness pioneered by companies such as Cambridge Cancer Genomics.

5. Balancing the economics and promise of personalised oncology

Even as our understanding of the heterogeneity in cancer makes it ever more a part of the need for personalised treatment strategies, and as our computational tools begin to make this possible, a significant barrier to adoption is becoming apparent: the cost of personalised medicine in oncology is increasing [76]. There exists a profound conflict at the heart of precision oncology between the varied and contrasting priorities of the pharmaceutical industry, local and national governments, international medical community, and patients, which needs to be reviewed and balanced. Even as the stated aims of each stakeholder align, individual incentive sets around target patient populations, the need to increase revenues and offset inefficiencies and the need to personalise treatment plans must be aligned if precision oncology is to become truly widespread.

It is no secret that the financial burden of cancer to the global economy is significant, perhaps more surprising is the personal economic costs. In the UK, where healthcare is free at the point of use, a cancer diagnosis results in a net loss to an individual of >£570, and in the US, a diagnosis increases the likelihood of bankruptcy by 250% [76]. Aside from direct costs associated with health insurance deductibles and co-pays (e.g. in the US) and ancillary spending (e.g. in the UK), cancer is among the most expensive diseases to manage across the healthcare ecosystem. In particular, the last decade or so has seen a substantial increase in the direct costs of cancer medicine. At the turn of the twenty-first century, the average annual cost of a new anti-cancer therapy was a little under $10,000, by 2016 this had risen to $100,000 for the same treatment duration [77]. Proponents of the pharmaceutical industry would point out that treatment modalities have increased in complexity significantly in the same period; however, there is little evidence that improvements in patient outcomes have kept pace with the increase in costs.

Indeed, when viewed in terms of Quality Adjusted Life Years (QALYs), the incremental gain from new treatment modalities such as targeted and antibody therapies launched between 1999 and 2011 is 0.25 QALYs [78]. To put this in context, the average cost per QALY in the UK across all treatments is £13,000 and the threshold for approving treatments not intended for oncology by the National Institute for Clinical Excellence (NICE) is £20,000–£30,000. Moreover, beyond the cost of the drug itself, new treatment modalities are also associated with ancillary costs, for example, in companion diagnostics, development costs, and relevant associated technology. Personalised oncology is often seen as a saving grace in terms of making the high-quality cancer care sustainable. However, it is vital to understand the cost drivers in the current management of cancer and how these may change in a world of widespread personalised treatment in order to improve or maintain value for money in the future of cancer care.

Fundamentally, in order to bias the QALY calculation in favour of cost-effectiveness, we must either (1) improve targeting of drugs to only those patients who receive clinical benefit or (2) ensure that efficiency of the drug development process increases, to avoid fixed R&D costs being spread over a smaller patient population. Therefore, if precision oncology has the potential of improving the efficacy of drug targeting, we must look to cost-saving efficiencies in the drug development process.

Clearly, a key driver of the increasing cost of cancer care is the reduction in R&D efficiency in pharmaceuticals companies; indeed, this is ingrained in our collective understanding of the industry that has even been dubbed 'Eroom's Law' [79]. It has long been argued that all the 'low hanging fruit' (i.e. all the easy targets) has long since been 'picked'. However, this assumption belittles the fact that of the $2.6 billion it costs to develop a new drug, a large proportion of this cost is associated with a 90% attrition rate in Phase II–Phase III trials [14]. Nevertheless, there is a real danger that the majority of recurrently mutated targets in cancer, for example EGFR, have already been targeted and any new therapies can only hope to provide incremental benefit beyond what has already been done. Thankfully, as new avenues of biology are explored, such as immune disruption by tumours, or new targeting modalities are discovered, new targets become available.

A potential avenue for improving the efficiency of drug development comes from considering manufacturing practices. The past two decades have seen a shift from small molecules to larger and more complicated biotherapies such as monoclonal antibodies. The manufacturing methods of biotherapies are considerably more complicated and expensive than traditional small molecule therapies, which could in part account for the increasing cost of the end product. However, the efficiency of manufacture of biopharmaceuticals has increased dramatically over the same period: with typical yields increasing from 1 to 2.5 g/l during the period 2001–2014 [80]. The complexity of manufacture also creates an additional barrier to entry for new drug manufacturers. There is a real concern that identical production process will not equate to identical products, this could protect against generic manufacturers entering the market as soon as the initial patient protection has lapsed. Indeed, regulators have introduced regulatory processes for so-called biosimilars much costlier and more involved than for generics for small molecules.

An alternative explanation for the rising cost of cancer drugs, and one that is perpetuated by the media, is based entirely on market forces: that is the cost of cancer drugs increases because that is what the market is willing to tolerate. Proponents point to Orphan Drugs developed in the early 2000s. Initially priced in excess of $100,000 a year, the initial price was protested but inevitably paid. In terms of economic theory, this was a signal to the market of price elasticity and the willingness to pay more for health [1]. Though comprised of well-meaning individuals, pharmaceutical companies are corporations with a legal obligation to maximise value for their shareholders. A slightly more palatable theory simply points to the reimbursement period: cancer is an acutely managed disease, treated for 6 months before the patient either recovers or, sadly, passes away. Unlike with chronic medications, therefore, the entire R&D costs of that drug must be paid back over a relatively short period of treatment time. This, of course, raises the effective price.

Clearly the balance of incentives in healthcare is a complicated problem. The danger is that precision oncology has the potential to increase some of these complications. If we are to see widespread adoption of more personalised medicine, then care must be taken to address inefficiencies in the pharmaceutical development process. Otherwise, governments and patients may be left with an unpalatable bill for marginally improved health outcomes.

6. Summary

The estimated global incidence of all cancer types in 2015 was 17.5 million [81]. Fourteen per cent of all deaths in 2005 were due to cancer, which increased to 16% in 2015 [82]. In combating cancer, we have created a global industry of research institutes, pharmaceutical companies and specialist hospitals. This industry is currently failing to keep up with the rising global cancer burden and suffers from unprecedented inefficiencies. To solve this problem, we must incorporate technologies such as ML into the clinical care pathway. It is our opinion that investment should be focussed on the development of predictive biomarkers for treatment outcome, which take account of tumour heterogeneity and evolution. If we are to beat cancer, we should begin to look at it as a highly heterogeneous and dynamic disease that requires a more sophisticated treatment paradigm. In particular, we must be cognisant of tumour evolution and develop biomarkers suitable for the growing field of adaptive oncology.

Tumour evolution has been a key conceptual framework in cancer biology since it was first put forth by Peter Nowell in 1976 [18]. The theory postulates that cancers arise from a single cell that has a selective advantage over its neighbours and that cancer can be understood based on the evolutionary principles of selection and adaptation originating from this ancestral cell. Over time, cells within the tumour continue to adapt and bestow on the tumour whole, specific traits described as the Hallmarks of Cancer [22, 83]. These ideas have been developed using many of the concepts first established in evolutionary biology [84, 85], considering cancer as a disease of multicellular organisms in constant balance between Darwinian selection acting on the level of a single cell and the need for coordination between multiple cells for the good of the organism [86, 87]. From this perspective, cancers occur when an individual cell behaves in an autonomous manner, escaping from the mechanisms in place to coordinate cell behaviour [88].

The classic model of carcinogenesis describes multiple, successive clonal expansions driven by the accumulation of genomic changes or 'mutations' that are preferentially selected by the tumour environment [89]. However, it is important to note that natural selection acts on phenotypes rather than genotypes. Indeed, selection can be transient, favouring a specific phenotype in response to fluctuating changes in microenvironment. Indeed, recent work has uncovered monogenetic clonal expansion of phenotypic clones responsible for tamoxifen resistance in breast cancer [90] and chemotherapeutic resistance in CRC PDX models [91, 92].

More broadly, tumour evolution and resultant heterogeneity have been linked to several clinically important facets of cancer [10, 93], but are currently underserved in terms of clinical translation. ML and the age of big biological data give us the necessary power to address this problem, and the clinical and the financial need is now.

DOI: http://dx.doi.org/10.5772/intechopen.93160

Author details

John W. Cassidy
The Old Schools, University of Cambridge, Cambridge, United Kingdom

*Address all correspondence to: john@ccg.ai

References

[1] Howard DH, Bach PB, Berndt ER, Conti RM. Pricing in the market for anticancer drugs. The Journal of Economic Perspectives. 2015;**29**(1):139-162

[2] Pollack A. Drug goes from $13.50 a tablet to $750, overnight - The New York Times. New York Times. [Internet]. 2015:1-4. Available from: http://www.nytimes.com/2015/09/21/business/a-huge-overnight-increase-in-a-drugs-price-raises-protests.html?_r=1

[3] Cassidy JW. Studying the clonal origins of drug resistance in human breast cancers. Cambridge University Press; 2019

[4] Heppner GH. Tumor heterogeneity. Cancer Research. 1984;**44**(6):2259-2265

[5] Brattain MG, Fine WD, Khaled FM, Thompson J, Brattain DE. Heterogeneity of malignant cells from a human colonic carcinoma. Cancer Research. 1981;**41**(5):1751-1756

[6] Danielson KG, Anderson LW, Hosick HL. Selection and characterization in culture of mammary tumor cells with distinctive growth properties in vivo. Cancer Research. 1980;**40**(6):1812-1819

[7] Barranco SC, Ho DHW, Drewinko B, Romsdahl MM, Humphrey RM. Differential sensitivities of human melanoma cells grown in vitro to arabinosylcytosine. Cancer Research. 1972;**32**(12):2733-2736

[8] Weinstein JN, Collisson EA, Mills GB, KRM S, Ozenberger BA, Ellrott K, et al. The cancer genome atlas pan-cancer analysis project. Nature Genetics. 2013;**45**:1113-1120

[9] Cole MP, Jones CTA, Todd IDH. A new anti-oestrogenic agent in late breast cancer an early clinical appraisal of ICI46474. British Journal of Cancer. 1971;**25**(2):270-275

[10] Curtis C, Shah SP, Chin SF, Turashvili G, Rueda OM, Dunning MJ, et al. The genomic and transcriptomic architecture of 2,000 breast tumours reveals novel subgroups. Nature. 2012;**486**(7403):346-352

[11] Chia SK, Bramwell VH, Tu D, Shepherd LE, Jiang S, Vickery T, et al. A 50-gene intrinsic subtype classifier for prognosis and prediction of benefit from adjuvant tamoxifen. Clinical Cancer Research. 2012;**18**(16):4465-4472

[12] Liu MC, Pitcher BN, Mardis ER, Davies SR, Friedman PN, Snider JE, et al. PAM50 gene signatures and breast cancer prognosis with adjuvant anthracycline-and taxane-based chemotherapy: Correlative analysis of C9741 (alliance). npj Breast Cancer. 2016;**2**(1):3-4

[13] Cassidy JW, Bruna A. Tumor heterogeneity. In: Patient Derived Tumor Xenograft Models: Promise, Potential and Practice. Academic Press; 2017. pp. 37-55

[14] New drug costs soar to $2.6 billion. Nature Biotechnology. 2014;**32**(12):1176-1176

[15] Taylor P. AstraZeneca. FierceBiotech. 2019:8

[16] Herper M. The truly staggering cost of inventing new drugs. Forbes. 2012:38. Available from: http://www.forbes.com/sites/matthewherper/2012/02/10/the-truly-staggering-cost-of-inventing-new-drugs/

[17] Cassidy JW, Caldas C, Bruna A. Maintaining tumor heterogeneity in

patient-derived tumor xenografts. Cancer Research. 2015:132

[18] Nowell PC. The clonal evolution of tumor cell populations. Science. October 1976;**194**(4260):23-28

[19] Vogelstein B, Fearon ER, Hamilton SR, Kern SE, Preisinger AC, Leppert M, et al. Genetic alterations during colorectal-tumor development. The New England Journal of Medicine. 1988;**319**(9):525-532

[20] Nik-Zainal S, Van Loo P, Wedge DC, Alexandrov LB, Greenman CD, Lau KW, et al. The life history of 21 breast cancers. Cell. 2012;**149**(5):994-1007

[21] Maley CC, Galipeau PC, Finley JC, Wongsurawat VJ, Li X, Sanchez CA, et al. Genetic clonal diversity predicts progression to esophageal adenocarcinoma. Nature Genetics. 2006;**38**(4):468-473

[22] Hanahan D, Weinberg RA. Hallmarks of cancer: The next generation. Cell. 2011;**144**:646-674

[23] Nik-Zainal S, Davies H, Staaf J, Ramakrishna M, Glodzik D, Zou X, et al. Landscape of somatic mutations in 560 breast cancer whole-genome sequences. Nature. 2016;**534**(7605):47-54

[24] Alexandrov LB, Nik-Zainal S, Wedge DC, Aparicio SAJR, Behjati S, Biankin AV, et al. Signatures of mutational processes in human cancer. Nature. 2013;**5**(12):134

[25] Martincorena I, Roshan A, Gerstung M, Ellis P, Van Loo P, McLaren S, et al. High burden and pervasive positive selection of somatic mutations in normal human skin. Science. 2015;**13**(2):432-456

[26] Martincorena I, Fowler JC, Wabik A, Lawson ARJ, Abascal F, Hall MWJ, et al. Somatic mutant clones colonize the human esophagus with age. Science. 2018;**34**(21):123

[27] Colom B, Alcolea MP, Piedrafita G, et al. Spatial competition shapes the dynamic mutational landscape of normal esophageal epithelium. Nature Genetics. 2020;**52**(6):604-614. DOI: 10.1038/s41588-020-0624-3

[28] Aparicio S, Caldas C. The implications of clonal genome evolution for cancer medicine. New England Journal of Medicine. 2013;**368**:842-851

[29] Weigelt B, Reis-Filho JS. Histological and molecular types of breast cancer: Is there a unifying taxonomy? Nature Reviews. Clinical Oncology. 2009;**6**:718-730

[30] Engels CC, Fontein DBY, Kuppen PJK, De Kruijf EM, Smit VTHBM, Nortier JWR, et al. Immunological subtypes in breast cancer are prognostic for invasive ductal but not for invasive lobular breast carcinoma. British Journal of Cancer. 2014;**111**(3):532-538

[31] Lal N, Beggs AD, Willcox BE, Middleton GW. An immunogenomic stratification of colorectal cancer: Implications for development of targeted immunotherapy. Oncoimmunology. 2015;**4**(3):1-9

[32] Gubin MM, Zhang X, Schuster H, Caron E, Ward JP, Noguchi T, et al. Checkpoint blockade cancer immunotherapy targets tumour-specific mutant antigens. Nature. 2014;**515**(7528):577-581

[33] Diaz LA, Williams RT, Wu J, Kinde I, Hecht JR, Berlin J, et al. The molecular evolution of acquired resistance to targeted EGFR blockade in colorectal cancers. Nature. 2012;**486**(7404):537-540

[34] Bhang HEC, Ruddy DA, Radhakrishna VK, Caushi JX, Zhao R, Hims MM, et al. Studying clonal dynamics in response to cancer therapy using high-complexity barcoding. Nature Medicine. 2015;**21**(5):440-448

[35] Bashashati A, Ha G, Tone A, Ding J, Prentice LM, Roth A, et al. Distinct evolutionary trajectories of primary high-grade serous ovarian cancers revealed through spatial mutational profiling. The Journal of Pathology. 2013;**231**(1):21-34

[36] Assenov Y, Brocks D, Gerhäuser C. Intratumor heterogeneity in epigenetic patterns. Seminars in Cancer Biology. 2018;**51**:12-21

[37] Almendro V, Cheng YK, Randles A, Itzkovitz S, Marusyk A, Ametller E, et al. Inference of tumor evolution during chemotherapy by computational modeling and in situ analysis of genetic and phenotypic cellular diversity. Cell Reports. 2014;**6**(3):514-527

[38] Sharma SV, Lee DY, Li B, Quinlan MP, Takahashi F, Maheswaran S, et al. A chromatin-mediated reversible drug-tolerant state in cancer cell subpopulations. Cell. 2010;**141**(1):69-80

[39] Andor N, Graham TA, Jansen M, Xia LC, Aktipis CA, Petritsch C, et al. Pan-cancer analysis of the extent and consequences of intratumor heterogeneity. Nature Medicine. 2016;**22**(1):105-113

[40] Misale S, Di Nicolantonio F, Sartore-Bianchi A, Siena S, Bardelli A. Resistance to anti-EGFR therapy in colorectal cancer: From heterogeneity to convergent evolution. Cancer Discovery. 2014;**4**:1269-1280

[41] Kostadinov R, Maley CC, Kuhner MK. Bulk genotyping of biopsies can create spurious evidence for hetereogeneity in mutation content. PLoS Computational Biology. 2016;**12**(4):1

[42] Jiang L, Chen H, Pinello L, Yuan GC. GiniClust: Detecting rare cell types from single-cell gene expression data with Gini index. Genome Biology. 2016;**17**(1):4-5

[43] Kennedy SR, Schmitt MW, Fox EJ, Kohrn BF, Salk JJ, Ahn EH, et al. Detecting ultralow-frequency mutations by duplex sequencing. Nature Protocols. 2014;**9**(11):2586-2606

[44] Wang Y, Waters J, Leung ML, Unruh A, Roh W, Shi X, et al. Clonal evolution in breast cancer revealed by single nucleus genome sequencing. Nature. 2014;**512**(7513):155-160

[45] Caravagna G, Giarratano Y, Ramazzotti D, Tomlinson I, Graham TA, Sanguinetti G, et al. Detecting repeated cancer evolution from multi-region tumor sequencing data. Nature Methods. 2018;**15**(9):707-714

[46] Dubourg-Felonneau G, Cannings T, Cotter F, Thompson H, Patel N, Cassidy JW, et al. A framework for implementing machine learning on omics data. Machine Learning for Health. 2018;**1**(1):3-10. Available from: http://arxiv.org/abs/1811.10455 [Accessed: 23 February 2020]

[47] Vamathevan J, Clark D, Czodrowski P, Dunham I, Ferran E, Lee G, et al. Applications of machine learning in drug discovery and development. Nature Reviews Drug Discovery. 2019:367

[48] Li B, Shin H, Gulbekyan G, Pustovalova O, Nikolsky Y, Hope A, et al. Development of a drug-response modeling framework to identify cell line derived translational biomarkers that can predict treatment outcome to Erlotinib or Sorafenib. PLoS One. 2015;**10**(6):23-48

[49] Van Gool AJ, Bietrix F, Caldenhoven E, Zatloukal K, Scherer A, Litton JE, et al. Bridging the translational innovation gap through good biomarker practice. Nature Reviews. Drug Discovery. 2017;**16**:587-588

[50] Kraus VB. Biomarkers as drug development tools: Discovery, validation, qualification and use. Nature Reviews Rheumatology. 2018;**14**:354-362

[51] Clifford HW, Cassidy AP, Vaughn C, Tsai ES, Seres B, Patel N, et al. Profiling lung adenocarcinoma by liquid biopsy: Can one size fit all? Cancer Nanotechnology. 2016;**6**(3):377

[52] Kim ES, Herbst RS, Wistuba II, Jack Lee J, Blumenschein GR, Tsao A, et al. The BATTLE trial: Personalizing therapy for lung cancer. Cancer Discovery. 2011;**3**(12):123-231

[53] Finn RS, Ryoo B-Y, Merle P, Kudo M, Bouattour M, Lim H-Y, et al. Results of KEYNOTE-240: Phase 3 study of pembrolizumab (Pembro) vs best supportive care (BSC) for second line therapy in advanced hepatocellular carcinoma (HCC). Journal of Clinical Oncology. 2019;**2**(1):395-414

[54] Shi L, Campbell G, Jones WD, Campagne F, Wen Z, Walker SJ, et al. The Microarray Quality Control (MAQC)-II study of common practices for the development and validation of microarray-based predictive models. Nature Biotechnology. 2010;**28**(8):827-838

[55] Zhan F, Huang Y, Colla S, Stewart JP, Hanamura I, Gupta S, et al. The molecular classification of multiple myeloma. Blood. 2006;**108**(6):2020-2028

[56] Shaughnessy JD, Zhan F, Burington BE, Huang Y, Colla S, Hanamura I, et al. Avalidated gene expression model of high-risk multiple myeloma is defined by deregulated expression of genes mapping to chromosome 1. Blood. 2007;**109**(6):2276-2284

[57] Zhan F, Barlogie B, Mulligan G, Shaughnessy JD, Bryant B. High-risk myeloma: A gene expression-based risk-stratification model for newly diagnosed multiple myeloma treated with high-dose therapy is predictive of outcome in relapsed disease treated with single-agent bortezomib or high-dose dexamethasone. Blood. 2008;**111**:968-969

[58] Decaux O, Lodé L, Magrangeas F, Charbonnel C, Gouraud W, Jézéquel P, et al. Prediction of survival in multiple myeloma based on gene expression profiles reveals cell cycle and chromosomal instability signatures in high-risk patients and hyperdiploid signatures in low-risk patients: A study of the Intergroupe Francophone du Myélom. Journal of Clinical Oncology. 2008;**26**(29):4798-4805

[59] Costello JC, Heiser LM, Georgii E, Gönen M, Menden MP, Wang NJ, et al. A community effort to assess and improve drug sensitivity prediction algorithms. Nature Biotechnology. 2014;**32**(12):1202-1212

[60] Rahman R, Otridge J, Pal R. IntegratedMRF: Random forest-based framework for integrating prediction from different data types. Bioinformatics. 2017;**33**(9):1407-1410

[61] Bunte K, Leppäaho E, Saarinen I, Kaski S. Sparse group factor analysis for biclustering of multiple data sources. Bioinformatics. 2016;**32**(16):2457-2463

[62] Huang C, Mezencev R, McDonald JF, Vannberg F. Open source machine-learning algorithms for the prediction of optimal cancer drug therapies. PLoS One. 2017;**12**(10):4

[63] Hejase HA, Chan C. Improving drug sensitivity prediction using different types of data. CPT: Pharmacometrics & Systems Pharmacology. 2015;**4**(2):98-105

[64] Dubourg-Felonneau G, Kussad Y, Kirkham D, Cassidy JW, Patel N, Clifford HW. Learning embeddings from cancer mutation sets for classification tasks. Machine Learning for Health. 2019;**3**(1):1-12. Available from: http://arxiv.org/abs/1911.09008 [Accessed: 23 February 2020]

[65] Cassidy JW, Batra AS, Greenwood W, Bruna A. Patient-derived tumour xenografts for breast cancer drug discovery. Endocrine-Related Cancer. 2016:5555

[66] Bruna A, Rueda OM, Greenwood W, Batra AS, Callari M, Batra RN, et al. A biobank of breast cancer explants with preserved intra-tumor heterogeneity to screen anticancer compounds. Cell. 2016;**167**(1):260.e22-274.e22

[67] Linton-Reid K, Clifford H, Thompson JS. Enhanced cancer subtyping via pan-transcriptomics data fusion, Monte-Carlo consensus clustering, and auto classifier creation. In: ACM International Conference Proceeding Series. 2019. DOI: 10.1101/2019.12.16.870188

[68] Paré G, Mao S, Deng WQ. A machine-learning heuristic to improve gene score prediction of polygenic traits. Scientific Reports. 2017;**12**(1):1234-1265

[69] Khera AV, Chaffin M, Aragam KG, Haas ME, Roselli C, Choi SH, et al. Genome-wide polygenic scores for common diseases identify individuals with risk equivalent to monogenic mutations. Nature Genetics. 2018:6593-6612

[70] Tasaki S, Suzuki K, Kassai Y, Takeshita M, Murota A, Kondo Y, et al. Multi-omics monitoring of drug response in rheumatoid arthritis in pursuit of molecular remission. Nature Communications. 2018;**2**(1):144

[71] Way GP, Greene CS. Extracting a biologically relevant latent space from cancer transcriptomes with variational autoencoders. In: Pacific Symposium on Biocomputing. 2018. p. 134

[72] Pallmann P, Bedding AW, Choodari-Oskooei B, Dimairo M, Flight L, Hampson LV, et al. Adaptive designs in clinical trials: Why use them, and how to run and report them. BMC Medicine. 2018:12-16

[73] Lattimore T, Szepesvari C. Bandit algorithms. Cambridge University Press. 2018;**23**(1):112-134

[74] Villar SS, Bowden J, Wason J. Multi-armed bandit models for the optimal design of clinical trials: Benefits and challenges. Statistical Science. 2015;**2**(1):234-254

[75] Armitage P. The search for optimality in clinical trials. International Statistical Review. 1985;**3**(3):2-12

[76] Flaum N, Hall P, McCabe C. Balancing the economics and ethics of personalised oncology. Trends in Cancer. 2018:14-34

[77] Luengo-Fernandez R, Leal J, Gray A, Sullivan R. Economic burden of cancer across the European Union: A population-based cost analysis. The Lancet Oncology. 2013;**43**(3):145

[78] Chambers JD, Thorat T, Pyo J, Chenoweth M, Neumann PJ. Despite high costs, specialty drugs may offer value for money comparable to that of traditional drugs. Health Affairs. 2014;**3**(5):35

[79] Van Norman GA. Overcoming the declining trends in innovation

and investment in cardiovascular therapeutics: Beyond EROOM's law. JACC: Basic to Translational Science. 2017;**12**(1):123

[80] Langer E, Rader R. Biopharmaceutical manufacturing: Historical and future trends in titers, yields, and efficiency in commercial-scale bioprocessing. Bioprocessing Journal. 2015;**3**(34):143

[81] Fitzmaurice C, Allen C, Barber RM, Barregard L, Bhutta ZA, Brenner H, et al. Global, regional, and national cancer incidence, mortality, years of life lost, years lived with disability, and disability-adjusted life-years for 32 cancer groups, 1990 to 2015: A systematic analysis for the Global Burden of Disease Study. JAMA Oncology. 2017;**3**:524-548

[82] Wang H, Naghavi M, Allen C, Barber RM, Bhutta ZA, Carter A, et al. Global, regional, and national life expectancy, all-cause mortality, and cause-specific mortality for 249 causes of death, 1980-2015: A systematic analysis for the Global Burden of Disease Study 2015. Lancet. 2016;**388**(10053):1459-1544

[83] Hanahan D, Weinberg RA. The hallmarks of cancer. Cell. 2000;**100**:57-70

[84] Pepper JW, Findlay CS, Kassen R, Spencer SL, Maley CC. Cancer research meets evolutionary biology. Evolutionary Applications. 2009;**2**(1):62-70

[85] Greaves M, Maley CC. Clonal evolution in cancer. Nature. 2012;**481**:306-313

[86] Merlo LMF, Pepper JW, Reid BJ, Maley CC. Cancer as an evolutionary and ecological process. Nature Reviews. Cancer. 2006;**6**:924-935

[87] Aktipis CA, Nesse RM. Evolutionary foundations for cancer biology. In: Evolutionary Applications. Vol. 6. Wiley/Blackwell; 2013. pp. 144-159

[88] Stratton MR, Campbell PJ, Futreal PA. The cancer genome. Nature. 2009;**458**:719-724

[89] Yates LR, Campbell PJ. Evolution of the cancer genome. Nature Reviews Genetics. 2012;**13**:795-806

[90] Patten DK, Corleone G, Győrffy B, Perone Y, Slaven N, Barozzi I, et al. Enhancer mapping uncovers phenotypic heterogeneity and evolution in patients with luminal breast cancer. Nature Medicine. 2018;**24**(9):1469-1480

[91] Kreso A, van Galen P, Pedley NM, Lima-Fernandes E, Frelin C, Davis T, et al. Self-renewal as a therapeutic target in human colorectal cancer. Nature Medicine. 2014;**20**(1):29-36

[92] Kreso A, O'Brien CA, Van Galen P, Gan OI, Notta F, Brown AMK, et al. Variable clonal repopulation dynamics influence chemotherapy response in colorectal cancer. Science. 2013;**339**(6119):543-548

[93] Shah SP, Roth A, Goya R, Oloumi A, Ha G, Zhao Y, et al. The clonal and mutational evolution spectrum of primary triple-negative breast cancers. Nature. 2012;**486**(7403):395-399

Chapter 6

Efficacy Evaluation in the Era of Precision Medicine: The Scope for AI

Dominic Magirr

Abstract

Patient stratification and the use of real-world evidence in regulatory decision-making are two key areas where algorithms are having an impact on drug development. The two are linked: increased patient stratification makes it harder to recruit patients into randomized-controlled trials, increasing the pressure on drug developers to find alternative sources of evidence for showing efficacy. In addition to real-world evidence, we are also seeing the emergence of more efficient 'master protocol trials', where multiple targeted agents can be evaluated simultaneously. In this chapter, I will review these developments and investigate the limitations for AI in terms of demonstrating the efficacy of novel targeted agents.

Keywords: drug development, precision medicine, statistics

1. Introduction

The use of algorithms to find patterns and make predictions from multiple data sources—here referred to as artificial intelligence (AI)—is having an increasingly large impact on clinical drug development.

Algorithms can be applied to combined clinical and genetic data sets to stratify patient populations into subgroups, based on shared characteristics or similar prognostic profiles [1–2]. This would appear to make sense, since the majority of new drugs approved by the US FDA in recent years have been targeted towards specific genetic aberrations [3–4]. If we increase our search, we will find more genetic aberrations, more drug targets, and more potentially efficacious drugs. However, this approach also presents severe challenges in the clinical stages of drug development, as the size, complexity and duration of studies increases.

One way to react to increased cost and duration is to improve the operational efficiency of clinical trials. The last decade has seen the emergence of 'master protocol trials', which allow several substudies to be conducted simultaneously, reducing the rate of screen failures [5]. In addition, there is increasing enthusiasm for augmenting (possibly even replacing) randomized-controlled trials (RCTs) with external and real-world data, where it is claimed that further use of algorithms can protect us from the biases that this approach would otherwise impose [1].

The purpose of this article is three-fold. Firstly, to explain how precision medicine presents challenges to traditional drug development, quantifying the effect of disease stratification on trial recruitment. Secondly, to describe how master

IntechOpen

protocol studies have emerged in response to these challenges. Finally, to explore whether it is possible for single-arm studies with 'synthetic control arms' to provide the same standard of evidence as a randomized controlled trial, thus reducing drug development timelines.

2. Disease stratification

Consider a patient population that can be stratified according to the value of a diagnostic test. The 'target' population consists of patients who test positive. The 'non-target' population consists of patients who do not test positive. Suppose that a new treatment is expected to be more effective in the target population than in the non-target population. Let θ^+ and let θ^- denote the treatment effect sizes in target and non-target populations, and γ denote the prevalence of the target group. Three things that we would like to demonstrate are:

1. Treatment benefit in the full population, $\gamma\theta^+ + (1-\gamma)\theta^- > 0$.

2. Treatment benefit in the target population, $\theta^+ > 0$.

3. Greater benefit in the target population than in the non-target population, $\theta^+ > \theta^-$.

Which of these is easiest to demonstrate, and which most difficult? To answer this, we compare the standardised statistics, Z, that we would use to test the corresponding null hypotheses. For most commonly-used clinical-trial endpoints, the test statistic ends up looking like

$$Z \sim N\left(\theta\sqrt{I}, 1\right), \tag{1}$$

where θ is the treatment effect size and I is the statistical *information*, which is typically proportional to the sample size [6, 7]. The *power* of a test is the probability that $Z > k$, for a threshold k, where k is chosen to ensure a given false-positive rate. The larger the expected value of Z, the higher the power. Therefore two trials ('A' and 'B') will have the same power if $\theta_A\sqrt{I_A} = \theta_B\sqrt{I_B}$, or, assuming that information is proportional to sample size, if

$$\theta_A\sqrt{N_A} = \theta_B\sqrt{N_B}. \tag{2}$$

We can use (2) to assess the relative difficulty of our three goals, firstly for the full population versus the interaction (1. versus 3.), and then for the full population versus the target population (1. versus 2.).

2.1 Full population versus interaction

It is shown in the appendix that a test of the interaction null hypothesis, $\theta^+ = \theta^-$, with total sample size N_{int}, will have the same power as the test for the full population null hypothesis, $\gamma\theta^+ + (1-\gamma)\theta^- = 0$, with sample size N, provided that

$$(\theta^+ - \theta^-)\sqrt{\gamma(1-\gamma)N_{\text{int}}} = \{\gamma\theta^+ + (1-\gamma)\theta^-\}\sqrt{N}. \tag{3}$$

For example, when $\theta^-/\theta^+ = 0.5$, for a prevalence of 50%, the ratio of sample sizes is $N^{int}/N = 9$. For a prevalence of 5%, $N^{int}/N \approx 23$. This shows how difficult it is to provide compelling evidence for treatment-biomarker interactions, and why drug development is still focussed on demonstrating average treatment effects. It is also explains why post-hoc data-driven subgroup identification following a clinical trial is often a bad idea. See Gelman [8] for further discussion.

2.2 Full population versus target population

A test for the full population null hypothesis with sample size N will have the same power as a test for the target population null hypothesis, $\theta^+ = 0$, with sample size N_T, provided that

$$\{\gamma\theta^+ + (1-\gamma)\theta^-\}\sqrt{N} = \theta^+\sqrt{N_T}, \tag{4}$$

or, equivalently, if

$$\frac{N_T}{N} = \left\{\gamma + (1-\gamma)\frac{\theta^-}{\theta^+}\right\}^2. \tag{5}$$

In (5), we have expressed the relative sample size, N_T/N, as a function of the relative efficacy, θ^-/θ^+ [9]. This relationship is drawn in solid lines in **Figure 1** for two potential prevalences (50% and 5%) when θ^-/θ^+ is between 0.5 and 1. For a prevalence of 50%, the targeted strategy requires up to 40% fewer patients than the non-targeted strategy. For a prevalence of 5%, a 70% reduction is possible. Note, however, that this is the relative number of patients *enrolled*. What about the

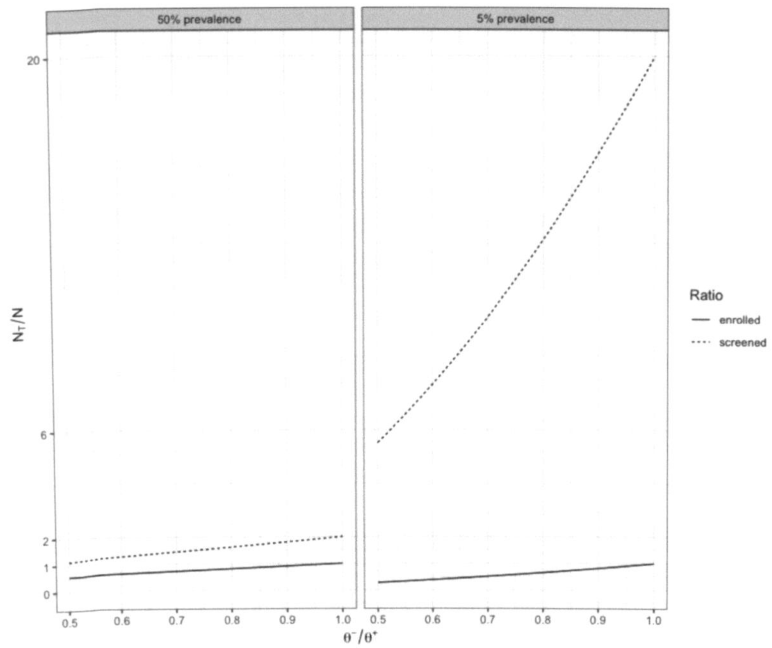

Figure 1.
Relative sample size when testing efficacy in the target population compared to the full population (N_T/N), *shown in solid lines. The dashed lines show the relative number of patients screened* ($(N_T/\gamma)/N$).

number of patients *screened*? In the full population the minimum number screened is N, whereas in the targeted population it is N_t divided by γ. The ratio, $(N_t/\gamma)/N$, is drawn in dashed lines in **Figure 1**. For the 50% prevalence case, there is a maximum 2-fold increase in the number screened for the targeted compared to the non-targeted trial. But for the 5% prevalence case, there is somewhere between a six-fold and a twenty-fold increase.

2.3 Situations where $\theta^- \ll \theta^+$

The conclusion from **Figure 1** is that population stratification is only likely to be useful if there exists a potential treatment where the treatment effect is considerably higher (e.g. at least two-fold) in the target subgroup than in the rest of the population. Marginal increases in efficacy are not enough in practice. The targeted approach would require a prohibitively large number of patients to be screened, compared to a trial in the full population which would have the same statistical power. Marginal increases are also difficult to establish empirically, as shown in Section 2.1. It follows that successful implementation of precision-medicine drug development is restricted to situations where there is strong biological and pre-clinical evidence for expecting $\theta^- \ll \theta^+$. Such cases certainly do exist, and the targeted trial is the only sensible approach here. Nevertheless, one still needs to screen a very high number of patients. This is expensive for the sponsor. It is also disheartening for patients who do not meet the eligibility criteria.

3. Master protocol trials

The high screen failure rate of precision-medicine trials can be mitigated to some extent by merging multiple sub-studies into a single 'master protocol'. The last decade has seen the emergence of the labels 'basket' and 'umbrella' to describe these complex studies. As a rule of thumb, a basket tends to refer to studies involving the same drug in multiple diseases, whereas umbrella is used when multiple experimental treatments are studied in the same disease. However, as reported by Janiaud and colleagues [10], these terms have not been applied consistently. Their systematic review of master protocol trials in oncology found 30 'basket' trials and 27 'umbrella' trials in a time period of 2006–2018, but with most studies starting after 2015. They explain that some basket trials are mistakenly labeled as umbrella trials, and vice-versa, but there are also trials that contain elements of both and thus become difficult to describe using current language.

Stallard and colleagues [11] propose a refined classification which replaces ambiguous labels with a more precise visual description, as shown in **Figure 2**. In each of the six designs, a small square is representative of a cohort of patients. On the left hand side are the basket-type designs, where there is only one new treatment (T) targeting a particular mutation (M), but this mutation occurs across diseases ($D_1, D_2, \ldots$). In the middle are the umbrella-type designs, where there are multiple treatments ($T_1, T_2, \ldots$) targeting particular mutations ($M_1, M_2, \ldots$), all within the same overall disease (D). The designs on the right hand side combine the features of the basket-type and umbrella-type designs. They allow for multiple disease types within each of the separate treatment-mutation combinations. Note, however, that it is always the mutation that is driving the choice of treatment, rather than the disease type. In all of the designs, for each T-M-D sub-study, it is possible to use a single-arm design (**Figure 2a**), or compare with a concurrent control arm (**Figure 2b**).

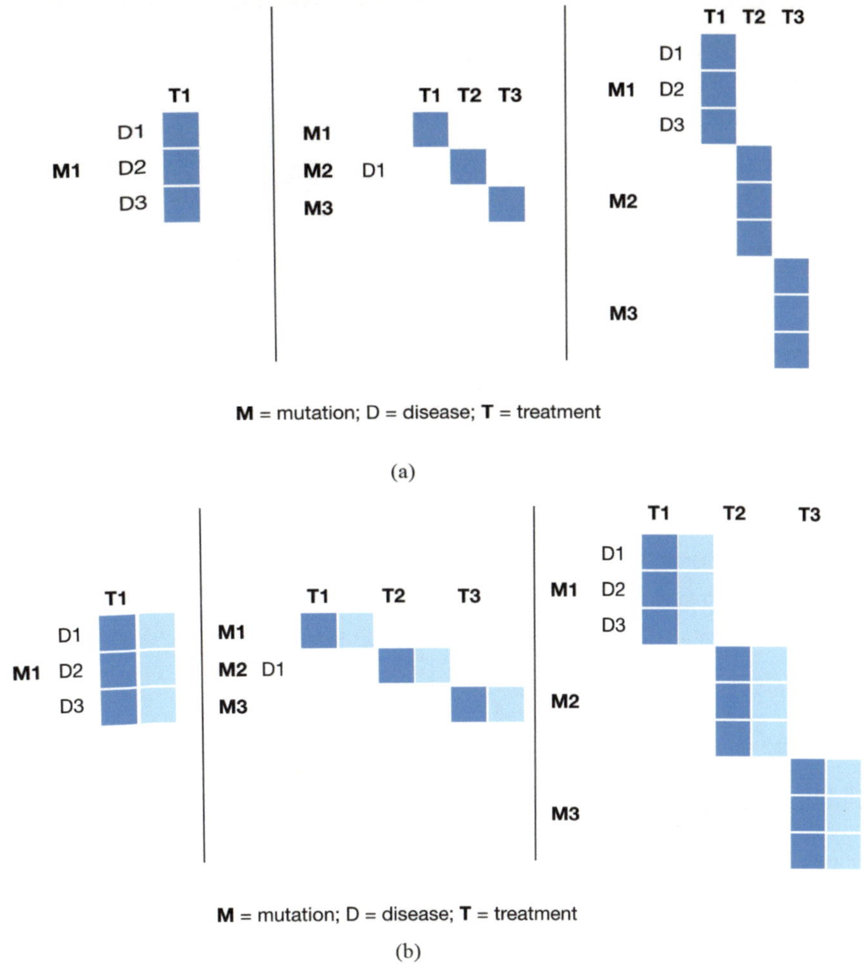

Figure 2.
A classification of master protocol designs by Stallard and colleagues [11]. Each square represents a cohort of patients. (a) Single-arm cohorts. (b) Concurrent control arms.

3.1 Example 1: Vemurafenib in cancers (not melanoma) with BRAF V600 mutations

Hyman and colleagues [12] report the results of a basket-type study with the same structure as the left-hand-side of **Figure 2a**. The treatment (T) was Vemurafenib, the mutation (M) was BRAF V600. There were several cohorts corresponding to different disease types (D):

- Colorectal cancer (CRC)
- Bile duct cancer
- Anaplastic thyroid cancer (ATC)
- Non-small cell lung cancer (NSCLC)
- Erdheim-Chester disease/Langerhans cell histiocytosis (ECD/LCH)

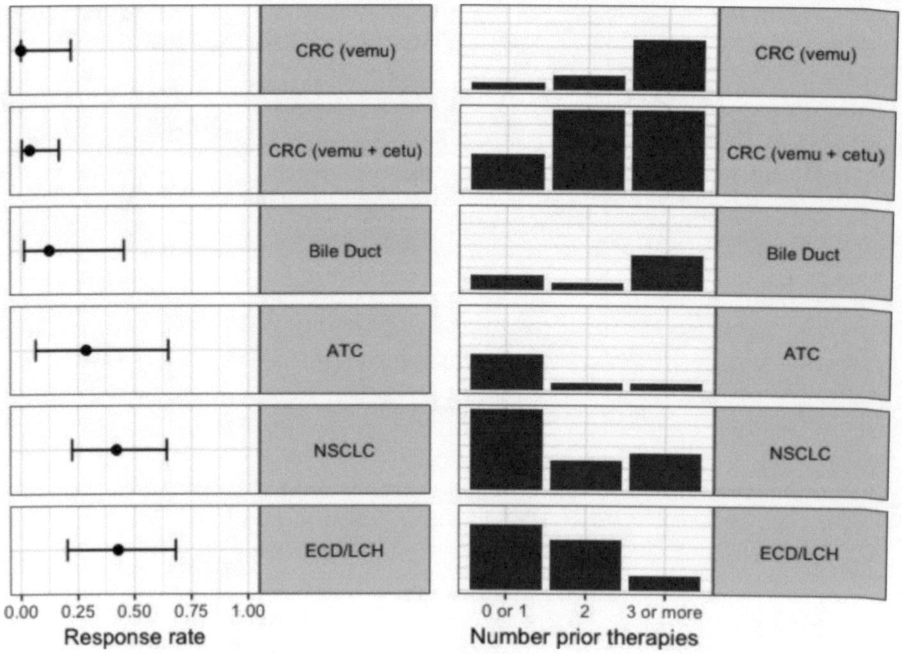

Figure 3.
Results from a basket-type study of Vemuarafenib [12–13].

A Simon's two-stage design [13] was used for each cohort independently to allow for early futility stopping. Consequently, the cohort sizes ranged from 5 to 27. Hobbs and colleagues [14], did a re-analysis of the data, and their findings are reproduced in **Figure 3**. Looking at the response rate across cohorts, it appears that there is more activity in NSCLC and ECD/LCH than in CRC. However, one can also see a clear inverse relationship between response rate and number of prior therapies, which muddies the water. This example highlights how difficult it can be to interpret uncontrolled studies.

3.2 Example 2: FOCUS4

An example of a master protocol trial that does include concurrent control arms is FOCUS4 [15], currently being run by the Medical Research Council Clinical Trials Unit in London. It has an umbrella-type design like **Figure 2b**. The disease setting (D) is advanced colorectal cancer. Mutations (M) include:

- BRAF mutations
- MSI deficient
- PIK3CA mutations
- Wild type

A centralised molecular analysis is performed on each patients tumor. Based on the results, patients are offered entry into an appropriate substudy, where they are randomized to receive either an experimental treatment (T) targeted to their mutation, or a control treatment.

The substudies will be analysed independently, as if they were separate trials. The big advantage over independent studies is the increased efficiency from the centralised molecular analysis, ensuring fewer screen failures. Complications may arise when patients are eligible for more than one substudy, and this has to be planned for in the protocol. Note also the inclusion of the Wild-type cohort in FOCUS4. This maximizes the proportion of patients who undergo screening who are given an option to go on a trial.

4. External control arms

Precision medicine is increasing the pressure on drug developers to find innovative ways to demonstrate efficacy without requiring ever larger and lengthier clinical trials. We have seen how operational efficiencies can be found in master protocol trials. A related development is the use of 'big data'—the bringing together of historical RCT data, electronic health records, advanced statistical modeling, and machine-learning—to produce a historical benchmark, or even a so-called 'synthetic control arm', that might allow a single-arm study to take the place of an RCT as a basis for seeking drug approval.

For this approach to be successful, the key use-case in oncology is a comparison of overall survival (OS). It is typical for inference to focus on the (log) hazard ratio,

$$\theta := \log \frac{\lambda_E(t)}{\lambda_C(t)}, \tag{6}$$

where it is assumed that the hazard of death on the experimental arm, $\lambda_E(t)$, is proportional to the hazard of death on the control arm, $\lambda_C(t)$, for all timepoints t. Another way to describe $\lambda(t)$ is that it is your risk of dying on day t given that you were alive at midnight. More stringent than proportional hazards is an assumption of constant hazards, $\lambda_j(t) = \lambda_j$ for all t $(j = E, C)$. Although an over-simplification, this model is often not a bad approximation to reality, and we will use it to compare operating characteristics for a two-arm RCT versus a single-arm trial with an external control arm.

4.1 Distribution of treatment effect estimators

The constant-hazards assumption allows us to express the log hazard ratio as the difference between the log-transformed median survival times,

$$\log \frac{\lambda_E}{\lambda_C} = \log m_C - \log m_E. \tag{7}$$

For a two-arm study with equal randomisation and D events, the estimate of the log hazard ratio has the following (approximate) distribution:

$$\hat{\theta} = \log \hat{m}_C - \log \hat{m}_E \sim N(\theta, 4/D). \tag{8}$$

If we were to run a single-arm study instead, but keep the overall sample size the same, i.e. put all patients who would have received the control treatment onto the experimental arm, we could use the test statistic

$$\hat{\theta}^* = \log m_C^* - \log \hat{m}_E \sim N(\theta + \log m_C^* - \log m_C, 1/D) \tag{9}$$

where m_C^* is our best pre-trial estimate for the median OS on the control arm.

4.2 Bias-variance trade-off

We can compare the precision of the two estimates in terms of their mean-squared-errors,

$$\begin{aligned} \text{mse}(\hat{\theta}) &= \text{var}(\hat{\theta}) + \text{bias}(\hat{\theta})^2 \\ &= 4/D + 0 \end{aligned} \tag{10}$$

and

$$\begin{aligned} \text{mse}\left(\hat{\theta}^*\right) &= \text{var}\left(\hat{\theta}^*\right) + \text{bias}\left(\hat{\theta}^*\right)^2 \\ &= 1/D + \left|\log m_C^* - \log m_C\right|^2. \end{aligned} \tag{11}$$

For low values of D, variance will be a bigger problem than bias. In this case, $\text{mse}\left(\hat{\theta}^*\right) < \text{mse}(\hat{\theta})$. However, as soon as

$$D > \frac{3}{\left|\log m_C^* - \log m_C\right|^2} \tag{12}$$

the bias will dominate, and the estimate from the two-arm trial will be more precise.

4.3 NSCLC example

What is a typical value for $|\log m_C^* - \log m_C|$? This depends on the context. The FDA have published data from 14 large randomized control trials [16] in advanced non-small-cell-lung cancer (NSCLC) conducted between 2003 and 2015. The median survival on the control arm across the studies is shown in **Figure 4**. Three of the studies were targeted towards patients with a particular biomarker. It is immediately obvious that these three data points are different from the rest, and this highlights the dangerous territory we are in. Nevertheless, if we focus on the 11 studies that did not use a targeted approach, the median overall survival ranged from 7 to 13 months. Taking an average value, a sensible choice for $\log m_C^*$ is $\log(9.5)$. We could also think about the 'true' $\log m_C$ for the current study belonging to the same distribution as the 11 other studies, which we might approximate with a normal distribution

$$\log m_C \sim N\left(\log m_C^* = \log(9.5), \sigma_{m_C}^2 = 0.03\right) \tag{13}$$

The expected value of $|\log m_C^* - \log m_C|$ according to (13) is $\sqrt{2/\pi}\sigma_{m_C} \approx 0.14$. Plugging this into (12), the two-arm trial would be more precise than the single-arm trial when $D > 153$.

4.4 Reducing the sample size

What if instead of moving patients from the control arm to the experimental arm and keeping total sample size the same, we run a single-arm study with half the number of patients, i.e. we keep the same sample size on the experimental arm and replace the control arm with an historical benchmark? In this case, the

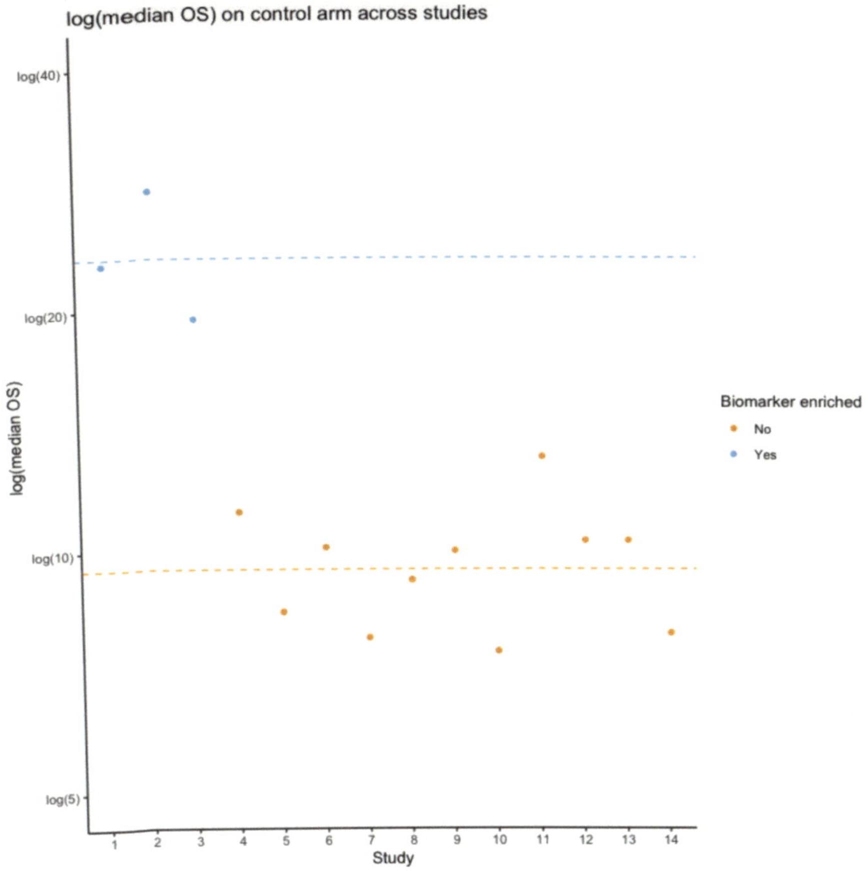

Figure 4.
Between-trial variability in median overall survival time from 14 phase 3 studies in advanced non-small-cell lung cancer trials submitted to the FDA [16].

mean-squared-error of the estimate from the two-arm trial will be lower than the single-arm equivalent as soon as

$$D > \frac{2}{\left|\log m_C^* - \log m_C\right|^2}, \tag{14}$$

where D is the number of events in the two-arm trial. For our lung cancer example, this would mean as soon as $D > 102$.

4.5 More advanced methods

In the previous example we were using the average value from 11 previous studies as a rather crude estimate of $\log m_C^*$. Is it possible to improve the precision using 'big data'—bringing together historical RCT data, electronic health records, advanced statistical modeling, and machine-learning?

We can look to a recent study by Carrigan and colleagues [17]. The group had access to individual patient data from 9 RCTs in advanced NSCLC conducted between 2011 and 2018, as well as electronic health records (EHR) from almost 50,000 patients. They used advanced regression and stratification techniques to estimate treatment effect sizes, and their results are reproduced on the left hand side of **Figure 5**. There is a high correlation (0.86) between the hazard ratio from

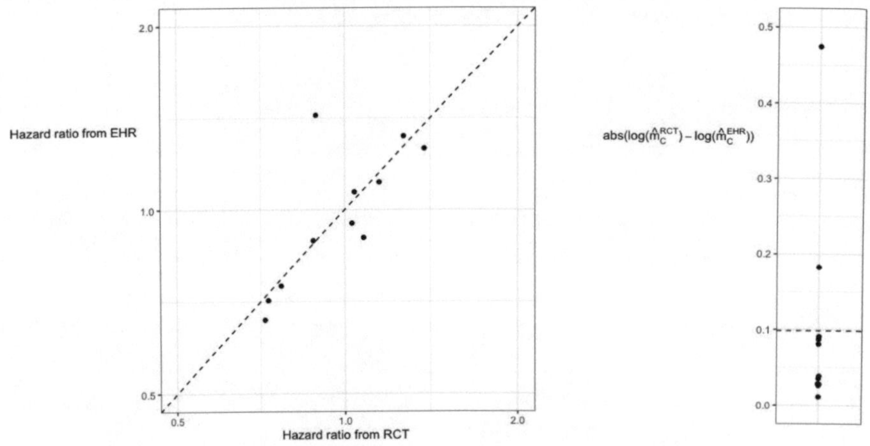

Figure 5.
Correlation between RCT-derived and EHR-derived hazard ratios from nine studies in advanced non-small-cell lung cancer [17]. On the right-hand-side, the results have been converted into an approximation of the bias when estimating the median survival time on the control arm using EHR data.

the RCTs and the hazard ratio that would have been observed had the control arm been replaced with electronic health record data. On the right hand side, the data points have been transformed into an estimate of the bias $|\log m_C^* - \log m_C|$, assuming constant hazards. The mean value is 0.1 and according to (12) this means that a two-arm trial would be more precise than a single-arm trial of the same total sample size whenever $D > 300$. Similarly, using (14), a two-arm trial will be more precise than a single-arm trial with half the sample size when $D > 200$.

To put these findings in some context, for a study with one-sided type-1 error of $\alpha = 0.025$, 300 events would give 90% power when HR = 0.69. Likewise, 100 events would give 90% power when HR = 0.52.

5. Conclusions

Advances in pattern-recognition and prediction algorithms have the potential to improve health outcomes, as well as making the drug development process more efficient. Nevertheless, it is important to have a strong grasp of some limiting factors, to avoiding spending time on futile endeavors.

The stratification of patient populations into ever finer subgroups is only likely to prove useful when there exist potential treatments with very large differential treatment effects. Marginal is not enough—it needs to be 100% more efficacious in the target subgroup than in the non-target subgroup. Otherwise, a clinical trial in the full population would have the same statistical power with far fewer patients screened. This means that we need strong biological rationale and robust pre-clinical evidence. In addition, it is essential that the diagnostic test has high sensitivity and specificity. Otherwise, a large treatment effect in the *true* biomarker-positive population would become diluted in the *observed* biomarker-positive population.

In cases where there is a strong rationale for a targeted approach, recruitment will be challenging. Master protocol trials can be an excellent option. They are an efficient way to test novel agents, and they increase the chance that a patient entering screening will be able to join a clinical trial.

Improvements in the quality of electronic health records, as well as better algorithms to interrogate this data, are a positive development that can enhance our understanding of health outcomes, and help enormously with clinical trial design and interpretation. Nevertheless, we should not forget the fundamental benefits of concurrent control [18], and should remain realistic about the ability of synthetic control arms to replace the real thing. We have seen that under favorable circumstances (highly prevalent disease, patient-level data from numerous high-quality large RCTs, tens of thousands of electronic health records, well-defined and accurately-measured primary endpoint, careful analysis), a single-arm study can provide similar precision to a two-arm randomized comparison with sample size in the low hundreds [17]. It is plausible, therefore, that for a new drug in this space with a very large treatment effect, a single-arm study may provide convincing evidence of efficacy. But one should expect this to be the exception, not the norm.

Conflict of interest

Dominic Magirr is an employee of Novartis Pharma AG.

Abbreviations

AI	artificial intelligence
FDA	Food & Drug Administration
RCT	randomized controlled trial
NSCLC	non-small-cell lung cancer
OS	overall survival
EHR	electronic health record

Appendix

Based on the test statistics (1) for the target and non-target populations,

$$Z^{+} \sim N\left(\theta^{+}\sqrt{\gamma I_{\text{int}}}, 1\right)$$

and

$$Z^{-} \sim N\left(\theta^{-}\sqrt{(1-\gamma) I_{\text{int}}}, 1\right),$$

we can define an interaction test statistic

$$Z^{\text{int}} := \sqrt{1-\gamma} Z^{+} - \sqrt{\gamma} Z^{-} \sim N\left(\left(\theta^{+} - \theta^{-}\right)\sqrt{\gamma(1-\gamma) I_{\text{int}}}, 1\right).$$

By (2), this test will have the same power as the full population test with sample size N if

$$\left(\theta^{+} - \theta^{-}\right)\sqrt{\gamma(1-\gamma) N_{\text{int}}} = \left\{\gamma\theta^{+} + (1-\gamma)\theta^{-}\right\}\sqrt{N}.$$

Author details

Dominic Magirr
Novartis Pharma AG, Basel, Switzerland

*Address all correspondence to: dominic.magirr@novartis.com

References

[1] Gao F, Wang W, Tan M, Zhu L, Zhang Y, Fessler E, et al. DeepCC: A novel deep learning-based framework for cancer molecular subtype classification. Oncogene. 2019;**8**(9):1-2. DOI: 10.1038/s41389-019-0157-8

[2] Bailey P, Chang DK, Nones K, Johns AL, Patch AM, Gingras MC, et al. Genomic analyses identify molecular subtypes of pancreatic cancer. Nature. 2016;**531**(7592):47. DOI: 10.1038/nature16965

[3] Shah P, Kendall F, Khozin S, Goosen R, Hu J, Laramie J, et al. Artificial intelligence and machine learning in clinical development: A translational perspective. npj Digital Medicine. 2019;**2**(1):69. DOI: 10.1038/s41746-019-0148-3

[4] FDA. Novel Drug Approvals for 2018. Available from: https://www.fda.gov/drugs/new-drugs-fda-cders-new-molecular-entities-and-new-therapeutic-biological-products/novel-drug-approvals-2018. 2018. [Accessed: 20 August 2019]

[5] Woodcock J, LaVange LM. Master protocols to study multiple therapies, multiple diseases, or both. New England Journal of Medicine. 2017;**377**(1):62-70. DOI: 10.1056/NEJMra1510062

[6] Whitehead J. The Design and Analysis of Sequential Clinical Trials. Chichester: John Wiley & Sons; 1997

[7] Jennison C, Turnbull BW. Group Sequential Methods with Applications to Clinical Trials. Boca Raton: Chapman and Hall/CRC; 1999. DOI: 10.1201/9780367805326

[8] Gelman A. You need 16 times the sample size to estimate an interaction than to estimate a main effect. In: Statistical Modeling, Causal Inference, and Social Science. 2018. Available from: https://statmodeling.stat.columbia.edu/2018/03/15/need-16-times-sample-size-estimate-interaction-estimate-main-effect/ [Accessed: 14 August 2019]

[9] Simon R. The use of genomics in clinical trial design. Clinical Cancer Research. 2008;**14**(19):5984-5993. DOI: 10.1158/1078-0432.CCR-07-4531

[10] Janiaud P, Serghiou S, Ioannidis JP. New clinical trial designs in the era of precision medicine: An overview of definitions, strengths, weaknesses and current use in oncology. Cancer Treatment Reviews. 2019;**73**:20-30. DOI: 10.1016/j.ctrv.2018.12.003

[11] Stallard N, Todd S, Parashar D, Kimani PK, Renfro LA. On the need to adjust for multiplicity in confirmatory clinical trials with master protocols. Annals of Oncology. 2019;**30**(4):506. DOI: 10.1093/annonc/mdz038

[12] Hyman DM, Puzanov I, Subbiah V, Faris JE, Chau I, Blay JY, et al. Vemurafenib in multiple nonmelanoma cancers with BRAF V600 mutations. New England Journal of Medicine. 2015;**373**(8):726-736. DOI: 10.1056/NEJMoa1502309

[13] Simon R. Optimal two-stage designs for phase II clinical trials. Controlled Clinical Trials. 1989;**10**(1):1-0. DOI: 10.1016/0197-2456(89)90015-9

[14] Hobbs BP, Kane MJ, Hong DS, Landin R. Statistical challenges posed by uncontrolled master protocols: Sensitivity analysis of the vemurafenib study. Annals of Oncology. 2018;**29**(12):2296-2301. DOI: 10.1093/annonc/mdy457

[15] Kaplan R, Maughan T, Crook A, Fisher D, Wilson R, Brown L, et al. Evaluating many treatments and biomarkers in oncology: A new design. Journal of Clinical Oncology: Official

Journal of the American Society of Clinical Oncology. 2013;**31**(36):4562

[16] Blumenthal GM, Karuri SW, Zhang H, Zhang L, Khozin S, Kazandjian D, et al. Overall response rate, progression-free survival, and overall survival with targeted and standard therapies in advanced nonsmall-cell lung cancer: US Food and Drug Administration trial-level and patient-level analyses. Journal of Clinical Oncology. 2015;**33**(9):1008. DOI: 10.1200/JCO.2014.59.0489

[17] Carrigan G, Whipple S, Capra WB, Taylor MD, Brown JS, Lu M, et al. Using electronic health records to derive control arms for early phase SingleArm lung Cancer trials: Proof of concept in randomized controlled trials. Clinical Pharmacology & Therapeutics. 2020; **107**(2):369-377. DOI: 10.1002/cpt.1586

[18] Senn S. Control in clinical trials. In: Data and Context in Statistics Education: Towards an Evidence-Based Society. Proceedings of the Eighth International Conference on Teaching Statistics (ICOTS8 2010 July). 2010. Available from: https://pdfs.semanticscholar.org/d36e/873d830932dd17c9ddf14e34dc542d14b63c.pdf [Accessed: 21 August 2019]

Chapter 7

AI Enabled Precision Medicine: Patient Stratification, Drug Repurposing and Combination Therapies

Steve Gardner, Sayoni Das and Krystyna Taylor

Abstract

Access to huge patient populations with well-characterized datasets, coupled with novel analytical methods, enables the stratification of complex diseases into multiple distinct forms. Patients can be accurately placed into distinguishable sub-groups that have different disease causes and influences. This offers huge promise for innovation in drug discovery, drug repurposing, and the delivery of more accurately personalized care to patients. Complex diseases such as cancer, dementia, and diabetes are caused by multiple genetic, epidemiological, and/or environmental factors. Understanding the detailed architecture of these diseases requires a new generation of analytical tools that can identify combinations of genomic and non-genomic features (disease signatures) that accurately distinguish the disease sub-groups. These sub-groups can be studied to find novel targets for drug discovery or repurposing, especially in the areas of unmet medical need and for selecting the best treatments available for an individual patient based on their personal genetic makeup, phenotype, and co-morbidities/co-prescriptions. This chapter describes new developments in combinatorial, multi-factorial analysis methods, and their application in patient stratification for complex diseases. Case studies are described in novel target discovery for a non-T2 asthma patient sub-group with distinct unmet medical need and in drug repurposing in a triple negative breast cancer population.

Keywords: precision medicine, genomics, patient stratification, target discovery, drug repurposing, therapy selection, clinical decision support, asthma, non-T2 asthma, cancer, triple negative breast cancer

1. Introduction

It is well-understood that the drugs available to and prescribed for patients, especially those with complex chronic diseases, are not always equally effective at treating their disease. In fact, many of the most widely prescribed drugs, including expensive on-patent medications, benefit only a small proportion of patients to whom they are prescribed [1]. There are multiple reasons for this including misdiagnosis, genetic variations in drug response/resistance, different responses at disease stages, ethnicity biases in clinical trials [2], and inappropriate reimbursement criteria for the disease.

Drugs are often prescribed on the basis of a defined clinical pathway that is guided by the diagnostic label given to a patient's disease in a 'one size fits all' approach. For highly heterogeneous diseases, this can seem like a largely trial and error basis before the right drug is found [3]. It can take months for patients to access a treatment that is effective and has a tolerable range of side effects. These delays not only waste drugs, they can increase the overall cost of treatment as a result of adverse events or worsening of the disease during the process of finding an effective prescription.

For example, it is notoriously difficult to select the right therapy and dose for patients newly diagnosed with depression. This is in part because depression is hard to diagnose precisely, due to it being multi-factorial, multi-genic with confounding situational influences and co-morbid with other conditions. As a result, depressive disorders are a huge societal burden affecting 6–7% of the workforce and costing the US economy $210 billion per year [4]. The failure to quickly access effective drugs requires multiple physician visits, resulting in lower quality of life and lost economic productivity for millions of patients. Many of the drugs that we do have are also poorly targeted 'sledgehammers' with widespread off-target effects affecting cognitive function, weight gain, sleep, and sexual function.

As a result of these challenges, UnitedHealth recently announced a new policy to use precision medicine for depression patients [5] in an attempt to escape the historical 'one size fits all' approach to medicine. Precision medicine attempts to use more personal information about the patients and more detailed insights into the disease to match the right drugs to the right patient.

Some patients may not even have available therapeutic options as none of the existing drugs prescribed on the clinical pathway for a given disease may work for them. This can leave pockets of poorly treated patient sub-groups and high unmet medical need. Such unmet needs exist in cancer due to the idiopathic nature of somatic mutations, but also even in relatively prevalent diseases with germline genetic predispositions such as asthma, diabetes and schizophrenia.

There are two methods of addressing both of these causes of unmet medical need. The first way is to try to identify new drug targets for pockets of unmet medical need within a patient population. This is effectively the traditional drug discovery approach, although it can be significantly enhanced by new AI-enabled precision medicine technologies.

The second approach is to try to predictively match existing drugs with patients who we have reason to believe will benefit from them. This is appropriate when we can see that those drugs are active at targets that we know are modulating disease processes inside a particular patient sub-group. This approach is called drug repurposing (or repositioning). Until now, many of the current repurposing examples prescribed in the clinic have been discovered in a serendipitous manner, but the advent of more detailed patient datasets and higher resolution patient stratification analytics tools enables us to do this systematically for all patients with a specific disease.

In turn, the knowledge of which drugs are likely to work for which patient sub-groups enables principled, evidence-led therapy selection in a clinical setting. Based on an understanding of the combination of factors driving a specific patient's disease, one or more drugs targeting those causative factors can be prescribed. This is better understood in oncology where mutational profiles have been used to evaluate the best therapeutic approach for specific tumours for many years. It also has application in other complex and chronic diseases whose aetiology, progression trajectory, phenotypes and therapy responses are mediated by multiple genetic and non-genetic factors.

These approaches, the tools and data that enable them, and the impacts that accurate patient stratification bring are discussed in this chapter.

2. Patient stratification: the key to delivering precision medicine

Precision medicine—providing the right drug at the right time to the right patient—promises to deliver better medicines, improved patient outcomes and lower healthcare costs. It has the potential to benefit millions of patients and save global healthcare systems tens or even hundreds of billions of dollars per year through new, better targeted therapeutic options, more accurate prescription, reduced over-medication, and better compliance.

Accurate patient stratification drives better understanding of the factors underpinning disease risk, rate of progression and therapy response, and presents us with a new palette of opportunities to impact patient care. Clinical decision support systems are beginning to apply patient stratification insights to inform treatment choices at the point of care. By increasing the chance that patients will get the right drug or combination of drugs first time, such precision medicine tools can reduce the cost of delivering care at the same time as maximizing patient benefit.

Expensive medicines or drugs with more severe side-effects can be reserved for those patients for whom all other cheaper and safer options have proven ineffective. This enables a more nuanced and personalized approach to prescription than allowed by traditional blockbuster or 'one-size fits all' approaches and overcomes some of the issues associated with the limited clinical efficacy of expensive novel therapies.

As described above, two approaches can be taken to delivering precision medicine. Either stratified disease sub-groups can be studied to find new targets for drug discovery, or the same detailed patient stratification information can be used to identify the best treatment (or set of treatments) from the existing formulary to apply to an individual patient given their genetic makeup, phenotype, co-morbidities and co-prescriptions.

Both approaches require a detailed understanding of the differential causes of diseases across a patient population. For monogenic diseases such as sickle cell anemia, Huntingdon's disease or cystic fibrosis, this is relatively simple, being very largely determined by a single pathogenic mutation, or in some cases different mutations in the same gene that have similar phenotypic effects. For complex, multi-factorial diseases such as cancer, dementia and diabetes this means finding combinations of features (disease signatures) that accurately describe disease subgroups rather than just finding single disease associated mutations in genes.

Revealing this level of detail requires a fundamental improvement in analytical tools. Disease population analytical methods such as Genome Wide Association Studies (GWAS) have attempted to find disease associated genes. They work by identifying single mutations (Single Nucleotide Polymorphisms or SNPs) that are over-represented in a case (disease) population compared to a control (non-disease) population and summing these signals to predict which genes might be most disease associated.

GWAS have found some new targets for some diseases, but in general their impact on drug discovery has been somewhat disappointing. In particular, GWAS have not lived up to the initial expectations that they would fully reveal the inherent complexity of multi-factorial diseases [6, 7]. Because they are designed only to find single SNP associations, GWAS cannot test the disease relevance of the huge number of potential combinations of SNPs, despite the fact that this is exactly what is driving differential disease risk, progression rates and therapy responses in patients. This has meant that GWAS can typically only explain a fraction of the observed phenotype variance and will only identify a portion of the targets that are relevant to a disease, particularly when these are most closely associated with one patient sub-group rather than the whole population.

A new generation of AI and multifactorial data analytics methods is now enabling us to start to untangle the complex combinatorial association signatures inherent in disease population datasets, properly characterizing disease sub-groups and identifying the different underlying factors causing and influencing their specific form of a disease.

One such tool, **precision**life **MARKERS,** is a massively scalable multi-omics association platform that enables the detection of high order epistatic interactions at a genome-wide study scale. It can find and statistically validate combinations of multiple (typically five or more) SNP genotypes (or other multi-omic features) that are found in many cases and relatively few controls, associating those combinations specifically with selected phenotypes, such as disease risk, progression rate and/or therapy response.

The insights generated provide a unique high-resolution insight into the architecture of complex diseases and evidence for the design and selection of therapy for individual patients. The importance of these tools to the delivery of precision medicine is described with example case studies in this chapter.

2.1 Combinatorial analysis tools for multi-factorial diseases

Precision medicine exploits (and is predicated on) the ability to identify more accurately which patients will respond to a specific drug or combination of drugs (and which patients will not). In cancer this principle is well understood even if the detailed associations between patient's mutations and their disease/response status are still being established.

There are clear genetic targets, such as BRCA1, BRCA2 and PIK3CA in breast cancer, KRAS in colorectal cancer, or BRAF or HER2 in several different tumour types. These typically result in (relatively) large effect sizes often driven by mutations in coding or direct gene expression control regions that result in significant loss of function in the targets. The causative principal is relatively clear in these cases, and patients with these types of cancers already have some personalized treatment options, and because the targets are identified, their diseases are the focus of even more detailed research.

However, outside of these coding region loss-of-function variants, other forms of cancer and other diseases, such as asthma, Alzheimer's, ALS and autism, are even more multi-factorial and heterogeneous. They often involve multiple disease causing and disease modifying factors from the genome, epigenome, immune system, epidemiological and environmental triggers, including diet and the patient's microbiome. In these diseases, multiple different disease related factors usually outside of the direct coding regions of genes accumulate and interact to exert the final phenotypic effect.

A specific patient's personal disease risks, rate of progression and responses to therapy vary enormously due to combinations of their mutations, predisposing phenotypic features and environmental influences. For these complex chronic diseases there are hundreds of features associated with different disease trajectories and therapy responses across the patient population.

The key to understanding diseases at a deeper level is to find combinations of these factors—disease signatures—that distinguish one patient sub-group from another. Using combinations of such factors provides a more granular way of stratifying patients, giving a higher resolution view of the disease. This enables novel, clinically relevant targets that were previously undetectable to be identified, providing a useful source of innovation for drug discovery/repurposing as well as informing therapy selection for individual patients (**Figure 1**).

The disease signatures can be used as patient stratification tools and form the basis of combinatorial risk prediction models as will be discussed later.

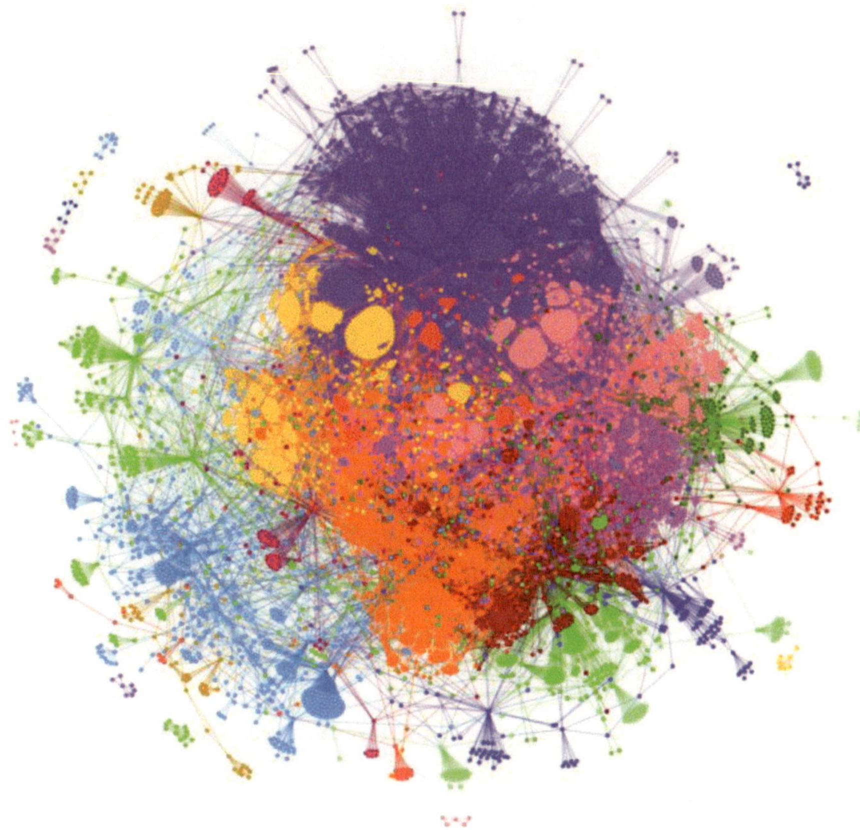

Figure 1.
Analysis of the disease associated SNPs in an 880 patient schizophrenia population (data provided by UK Biobank, combinatorial analysis performed by ***precisionlife MARKERS****, visualization using R Shiny). The SNPs are clustered and coloured to show communities of patients that share combinations of disease co-associated SNPs. This graph therefore shows both the key patient sub-groups as well as the combination of SNPs (disease signatures) that are associated with their specific form of the disease.*

2.2 Explaining mechanism of action and disease risk with combinatorial disease signatures

Knowing that a specific combination of SNPs/genes is strongly disease associated also helps to explain the metabolic context and the functional role those genes play in the disease. This information can be used to generate a minimally complex metabolic graph that connects the functions of all the genes contained in this network, as shown in **Figure 2**. This provides much more information about the context in which SNPs and genes occur than a standard GWAS study and enables focused validation of the metabolic role and disease relevance of the key targets.

Such signatures provide strong, testable hypotheses for the mechanism of action and also inform and accelerate the *in vitro* and *in vivo* target validation studies. This is a key contributor cited by AstraZeneca, GSK and AbbVie in improving their R&D productivity [8–10].

For the protective effect signature shown in **Figure 2**, it can be hypothesized that these genes all converge at a central signalling hub involving the insulin receptor (*INSR*), epidermal growth factor receptor (*EGFR*) and *PI3K* signalling cascade. Mutations in gene 6 appear to be modulating (blockading) the action of *INSR*, which is an important activator of *PI3K*, a key oncogene [11]. The PI3K/Akt signalling pathway is involved in a variety of processes such as cell growth and survival

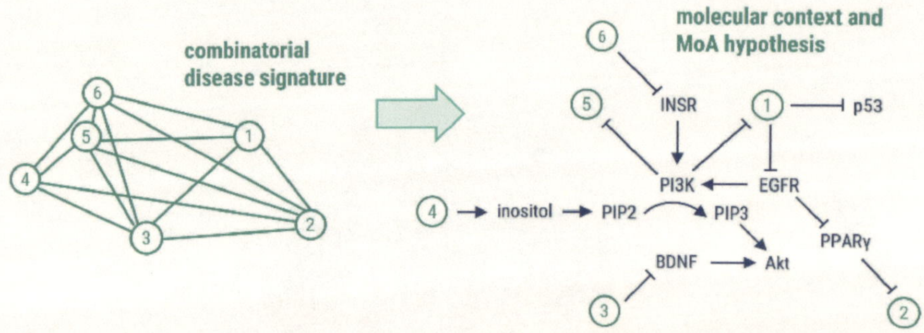

Figure 2.
Example of a 6 SNP disease signature associated with significantly reduced risk of developing breast cancer in a BRCA2 *positive population. This disease signature occurs in 145 people who have not developed breast cancer by the age of 55 and zero early onset (<40 years) breast cancer patients in a 1600 patient population.*

that are necessary for cancer progression [12]. If activation of PI3K is significantly reduced it would act to reduce oncogenesis, which would explain the lack of breast cancer in this sub-group even when their *BRCA2* tumour suppression capabilities are compromised by mutation.

The protective effect disease signature shown in **Figure 2** is just one of 3045 disease signatures identified from a **precision**life **MARKERS** analysis of the (germline) genotypes of the *BRCA2* positive population. Detailed patient stratification can be achieved by merging all of the disease signatures found in a study. Overlaying shared SNPs from the disease signatures and then clustering them by the patients in which they co-occur reveals an unprecedented view of the disease architecture in the population under study. For the first time, this type of analysis shows in detail the disease sub-groups and the combinations of SNPs associated with their specific form of the disease.

Figure 3 shows a merged view of the 3045 disease signatures identified in the *BRCA2* positive population described above. There are 762 unique SNPs in this set. Each circle on the graph below represents a single SNP with size proportional to its odds ratio (evaluated independently). Links connect SNPs that co-occur in cases and distance is inversely proportional to the number of shared cases. SNPs for the few (three) genes found by standard GWAS (*FGFR2*, *CCDC170* and *CCDC91*) are shown coloured red, yellow or green. Novel disease associated SNPs that can only be identified using a combinatorial approach are shown in grey.

This type of multiple clustering within a single disease is consistent even within very highly genetically determined diseases. In several studies, multiple non-overlapping patient sub-groups have been identified, including in bipolar disease [13] and diabetes [14].

Combinatorial analysis methods give novel, high-resolution insights into the disease architecture, enabling an understanding of how well a particular patient sub-population maps to the targets of drugs approved for the disease. Patient sub-groups with all grey SNPs on this view are much less likely to be responsive to drugs acting at the targets whose SNPs are coloured. For a given patient, their specific combination of SNPs will in large part determine which drug or combination of drugs are likely to benefit them personally. This detailed stratification is therefore a key enabler of precision medicine and the selection of personalized treatment regimens.

Such stratification also enables systematic identification of the drug repurposing opportunities for a disease. SNPs associated with targets of on-market drugs approved for other diseases can be mapped onto the disease sub-populations to identify and prioritize repurposing targets. This application will be discussed later in the chapter.

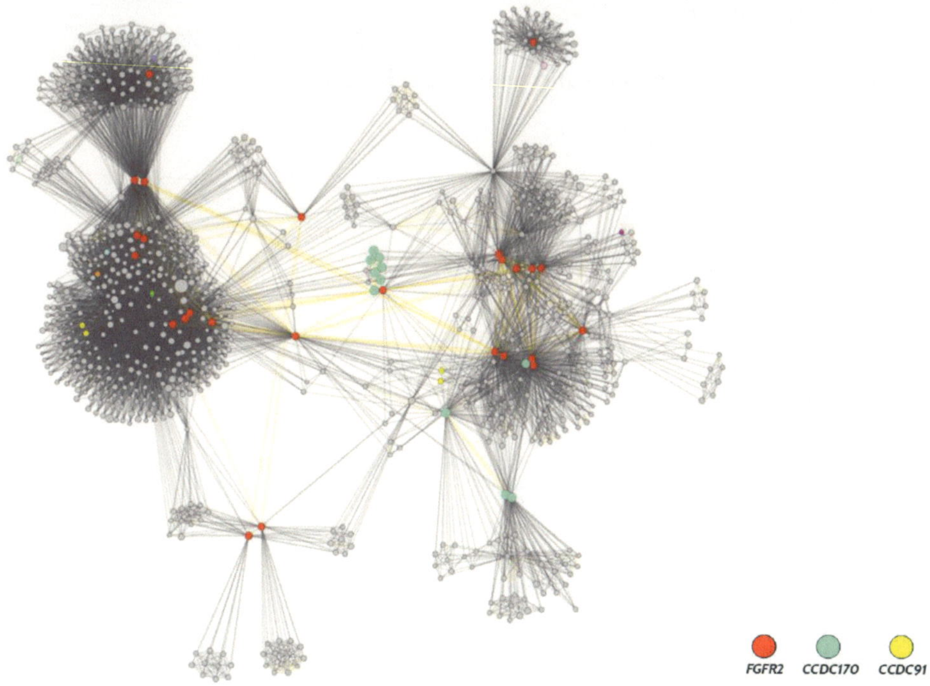

Figure 3.
Multifactorial analysis finds multiple new mutations and targets associated with disease risk in BRCA2 *positive breast cancer. SNPs are clustered by co-occurrence in patient cases—closer SNPs co-occur more frequently in cases. Yellow lines indicate that SNPs are in linkage disequilibrium.*

2.3 Evolution of genomic and other patient data sources

The key requirement for combinatorial analysis (and patient stratification) is a high-resolution view of the causes of a disease and how these are distributed throughout the patient population. This clearly starts with a well-diagnosed patient (and matched control) population with detailed molecular, phenotypic and clinical data. Because most diseases are multi-factorial and heterogeneous we usually need hundreds or thousands of patients' data in order to unravel the complex causes of disease. Such large high-quality patient datasets are beginning to become available with projects such as UK Biobank [15], disease charity projects such as Project MinE [16] in ALS, integrated hospital EMR systems and even pharmaceutical companies' own clinical trials datasets.

Over the past 10 years, the evolution of clinical and research data capture has progressed rapidly, led by huge progress in DNA sequencing technologies. It is well-known that the cost and accuracy of DNA sequencing has improved considerably more rapidly than Moore's law for computing. At the same time other data capture technologies have also been improving rapidly. There is now often a vast quantity of patient-related data available that can also be analyzed alongside genomics data to better inform patient stratification and clinical decision making:

- Omics data, including:
    - Proteomic and metabolomic data including liquid biopsies
    - Epigenetic data

- Patient clinical data
    - Prescription, progression and response information
    - Patient records
    - Claims databases
    - Longitudinal studies
- Epidemiological and hyper-local datasets
    - Lifestyle, diet and exercise levels
    - Environmental data on weather, dust, pollution and other stressors
- Microbiomic and metagenomic data from the patient and their environment
- Biomedical imaging and AI-derived feature analysis
- Digital biomarkers, including:
    - Active sensor-derived data from ambulatory monitors, mobile, and wearable devices
    - Passive environmental monitoring systems

Given that diseases are influenced by some or all of the non-genomic factors described above it is clear that in order to predict and explain the various forms of such diseases, we must be able to include all of these dimensions of data in our analyses. Using **precision**life **MARKERS** this can be done either as input variables in the mining phases, e.g. to find genetic signatures specifically associated with high BMI, high drinking cohorts of breast cancer sufferers, or as cluster variables after the analysis to validate and/or explain the genetic signatures identified.

The protective effect signature observed in **Figure 2** for example is known to be almost exclusively present in women of Hispanic ethnicity. In a standard GWAS, this type of population structure effect would have been deemed an artifact or confounder and eliminated using covariance methods. However, the protective effect is real and has a strong causative explanation, rather than just being a coincidental observation. This has real clinical relevance when women with that signature are considering their therapeutic and surgical options after having undergone a *BRCA* test.

3. Novel target discovery and validation

Effective drug discovery requires an understanding of many aspects of the disease. It is highly advantageous to have:

- A defined unmet medical need with freedom to operate and a clear competitive positioning

- A genetic explanation and testable hypothesis for the mechanism of action of the target
- Proof of differential expression of the target in disease related tissues
- Good chemical starting points with the right safety, bioavailability and off-target effect profile
- Accurate patient stratification biomarkers

This is the 5Rs framework of drug discovery as described variously by AstraZeneca, GSK and AbbVie [8–10]. Following these criteria has been shown to improve the chance of successful development of a program from inception to Phase III by over four-fold. These are clearly useful guidelines and heuristics that we can use to apply to the selection of novel targets following identification of unmet medical needs and stratifying patients accordingly. An example of how we use our pipeline to identify novel targets is described below using data from an asthma population.

3.1 Stratifying an asthma patient population into two molecular phenotypes

Asthma is a debilitating disease that affects 1 in 13 people. 5.4 million people are currently receiving asthma treatment in the UK [17]. Asthma patients can be categorized into two molecular phenotypes: those with high T-helper cell type 2 (T2/eosinophil) expression, which can result in an excessive inflammatory response, and those without (non-T2).

The aetiology of T2 asthma involves activation of the Th2 cells, which result in the release of cytokines such as IL-5 and IL-13. In turn, these cytokines recruit eosinophils to the affected tissue to counter the antigen(s) that triggered the Th2 system. Patients with a T2 phenotype currently have a range of targeted biologic treatment options available to them.

However, non-T2 patients lack such targeted drugs and often have to rely on conventional symptomatic control therapies (such as bronchodilators and inhaled corticosteroids), which do little to combat the underlying disease pathology. These non-T2 patients make up approximately 30% of the asthma population [18], meaning there is still a distinct clinical need for the development of novel targets for therapies that are targeted towards them.

While there have been many GWAS studies on asthma to date, prior studies have not focused on the genetic differences between T2 and non-T2 forms of asthma [19]. Our understanding of the genetics of T2 asthma are largely based on studies of the Th2-cytokine pathways.

Using **precision**life **MARKERS** with UK Biobank data, we performed a comparative study using a genotype dataset derived from UK Biobank to compare T2/non-T2 asthma patient populations. We used a slightly modified version of the case selection criteria presented by Ferreira et al. [20]. While UK Biobank does not have data from sputum samples, blood eosinophil counts are considered a good indicator of eosinophilia in the airways [21]. Using these criteria, we identified a total of 42,205 total asthma cases. We randomly selected 90,034 age- and gender-matched subjects from the same database to serve as controls.

We selected a total of 15,071 cases with serum eosinophil counts of 0.15 (1500 cells/mm^3) or less as the non-T2 cohort, and a total of 7094 cases with serum eosinophil counts of 0.35 (3500 cells/mm^3) or more as the T2 cohort. As some asthma cases did not have any eosinophil counts recorded, we excluded them from either group. In order to reduce errors due to misclassification, we also excluded a large group of cases with eosinophil counts between 0.15 and 0.35 which we considered to be moderate or borderline values.

Finally, we selected an age- and gender-matched control cohort of 21,688 subjects without asthma or similar respiratory disease. After quality control filtering, the genotype dataset included 547,147 SNPs for each case and control subject.

Our aim was to identify significant genotype differences between T2 and non-T2 asthma, to explain the observed difference in T2 phenotype and use this to develop novel targets specific for the non-T2 population. While UK Biobank does not have data from sputum samples, blood eosinophil counts are considered a good indicator of eosinophilia in the airways [21]. Therefore, we used blood eosinophil counts from the UK Biobank database to separate asthma cases into T2 vs. non-T2 cohorts.

Using **precision**life **MARKERS**, we performed several studies comparing the T2 cohort to the non-T2 cohort, and both cohorts independently to healthy controls. Firstly, we compared the lists of 'critical' SNPs with the lowest *p*-values from two of the studies: T2 vs. controls, and non-T2 vs. controls. We expected this comparison to identify three sets of critical SNP genotypes:

1. those that are significantly present in T2 asthma

2. those that are significantly present in non-T2 asthma

3. those that are common to both subtypes.

Figure 4 illustrates the numbers of critical SNP genotypes that are significant in each of these categories, indicating clear differences in SNPs between T2 and non-T2 cases.

The unique SNPs identified in the replication study (that is, those that show up in both cohorts as statistically significant minor alleles) follow a striking pattern. When prioritized by *p*-value, we see a large number of SNPs that relate to immune system disorders and asthma—which confirms our hypothesis that our analysis is finding biologically relevant high-order combinations of genotypic features.

We then mapped these SNPs into genes within +/− 1 KB and plotted the corresponding genes in a network diagram to illustrate the genetic differentiation of the two subtypes of asthma at the level of genes (**Figure 5**).

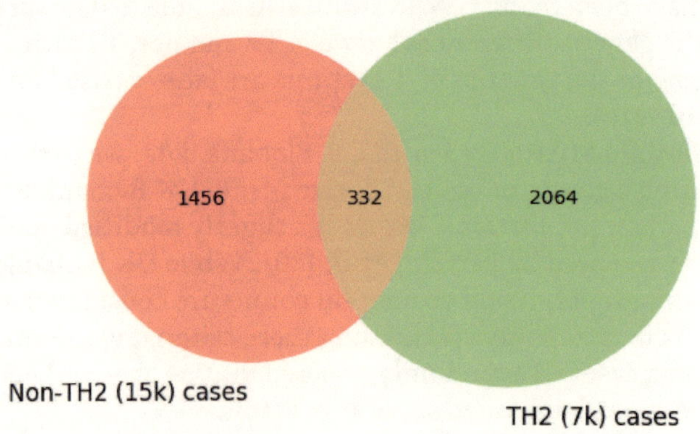

Figure 4.
Critical SNP genotypes that are significantly represented in T2 asthma (2064) vs. non-T2 asthma (1456) vs. those that are common to both subtypes (332).

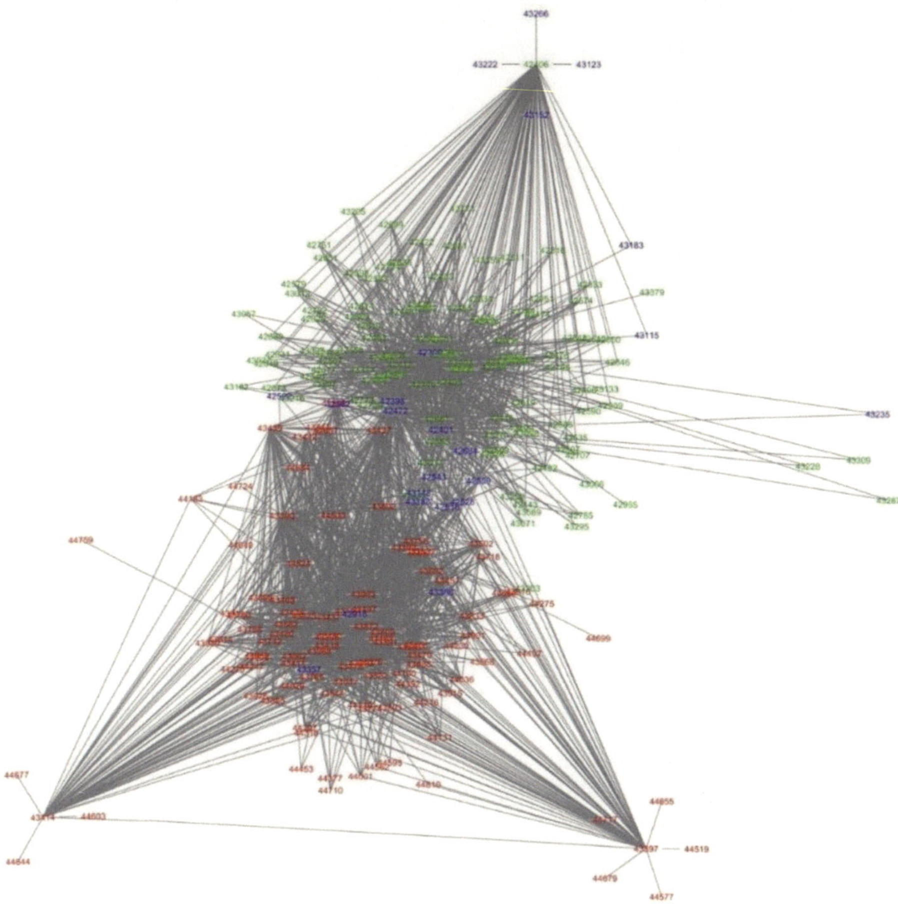

Figure 5.
Cytoscape plot illustrating major genes involved in asthma disease architecture. Genes in red are prominently involved in T2 asthma, genes in green are prominently involved in non-T2 asthma, and genes in blue are involved in both subtypes.

3.2 Using stratification insights to develop novel targets for non-T2 asthma patients

Next, we mapped the prominent SNP genotypes in T2 and non-T2 asthma to gene sets and performed a comparative pathway enrichment analysis (see **Figure 6**). As expected, the pathway enrichment analysis shows that T2 and non-T2 asthma are quite different diseases that share a common symptomatology but little else. This is at odds with the clinical prescribing pathways in place for asthma currently and indicates the need for the development of novel drugs that are specific for each patient sub-group.

While many of the most significant genes we identified in the T2 asthma population corresponded to classic T2-driven immune pathways, we identified a range of different non-immune pathways that were significant in the non-T2 cohort, including metabolic and neuronal mechanisms.

Several of the most significant genes in the non-T2 population encode enzymes that are involved in key stages of fatty acid synthesis and oxidation pathways. Although all the genes we identified represent novel asthma targets, both of these pathways have been implicated in driving asthma pathogenesis [22, 23]. We also

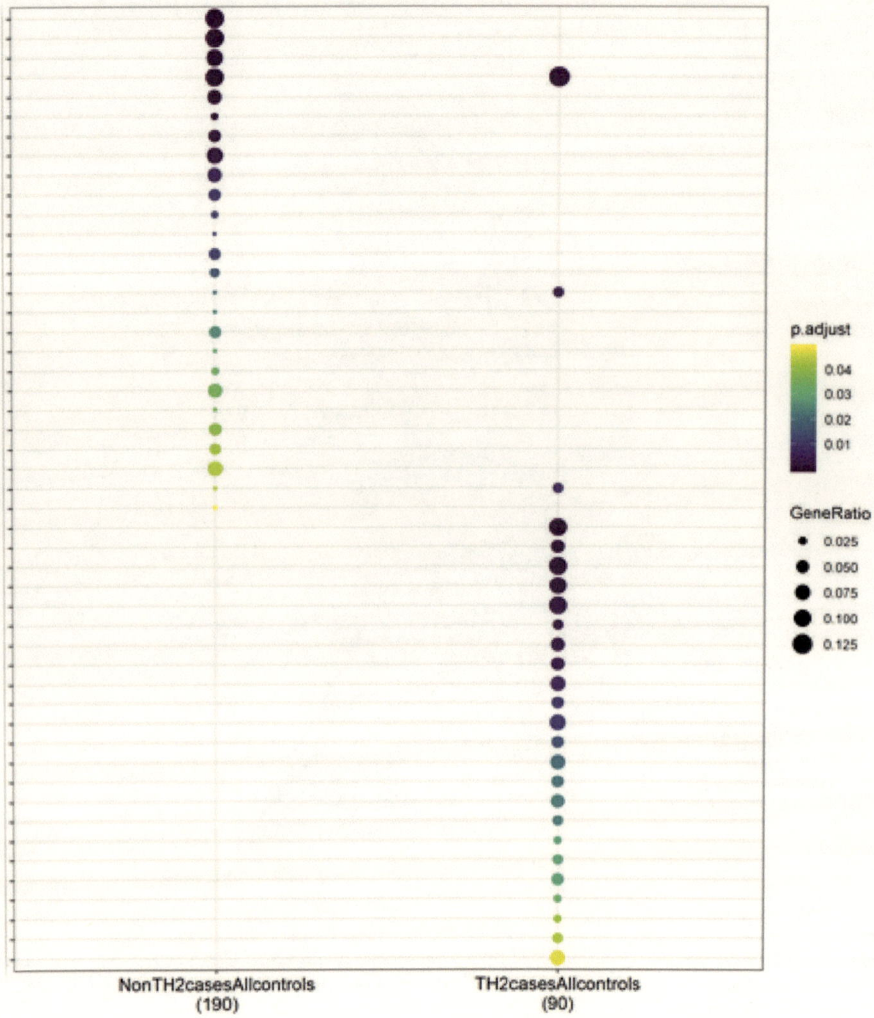

Figure 6.
Pathway enrichment results for T2 (right) vs. non-T2 asthma (left) showing distinct genes and pathways associated with the two forms of asthma (calculated using the ClusterProfiler R package).

identified targets that are involved in the promotion of LDL oxidation. Increased oxidized LDLs (oxdLDLs) are hypothesized to increase bronchial inflammation through recruitment and degranulation of neutrophils [24], and inhibitors of this pathway are already of interest to several pharmaceutical companies as potential new asthma therapies.

Furthermore, we found a range of genes that modulate several different neuronal pathways, including regulation of GABAergic transmission, purinergic receptor activation and glutamate signalling. This implies that non-allergic asthma is driven by a variety of different mechanisms that are not directly related to the immune system. None of the current biologic treatment options address these non-immune mechanisms.

The clear differences between the T2 and non-T2 asthma cohorts hold significant potential for better patient stratification, diagnosis and development of new treatment options. We have now identified over 20 novel genes that are significant only in the non-T2 population with strong, testable hypotheses for their mechanism of action. These represent promising opportunities for the development of personalized therapies for patients presenting with nonallergic asthma.

4. Systematic drug repurposing

Healthcare is a huge and steadily rising cost for all major global economies. Decades of dedicated scientific endeavor and extensive industry investment in biopharmaceutical R&D have paid huge dividends in improving the health of nations. The associated costs are however significant and are becoming potentially unsustainable [25] due to changing demographics, reduced R&D productivity and increasing use of expensive new treatment modalities.

A new way of routinely identifying the most appropriate and cost-effective treatments for individual patients is needed. This would identify the best, most personalized therapies from both the existing formulary as well as innovative new drug options to improve outcomes and lower costs. This is the compelling proposition underpinning precision medicine, and it is being enabled in oncology and beyond by new developments in AI technology aimed at improving patient stratification, drug repurposing and therapy selection.

Precision medicine promises to deliver better medicines, improved patient outcomes, and lower healthcare costs [26]. Personalized therapies can reduce costs associated with the inefficiencies of the 'one size fits all' approach of healthcare systems such as trial-and error dosing, hospitalizations due to adverse drug reactions, and reactive treatment [27]. However, developing novel targeted therapies for each patient sub-group is challenging. Robustly identifying disease causative mutations with druggable targets and developing the new medicines to target these is an expensive and time-consuming process that has proved difficult to scale, even with the advent of genomic medicine.

A more cost-effective approach can be to identify targets associated with the clinically relevant subgroups of patients with unmet medical needs and then search the current formulary to find the drugs that will be effective for each of them. This approach is called drug repurposing or repositioning.

4.1 Pharmacoeconomic pressures and healthcare costs

Over the last 70 years, improved vaccines, antibiotics, drugs and other healthcare interventions have delivered decades of profound positive change in lifespan, patient outcomes and socioeconomic productivity. But these benefits have come at a cost. In 2017, US healthcare spending was over $3.5 trillion—equivalent to $10,739 per person or 18% of the country's gross domestic product (GDP) [28]. This is expected to rise to almost $6 trillion (19.4% of GDP) by 2027 [29].

The world pharmaceutical market was worth $935 billion in 2017 [30]. 10% of the US healthcare budget is spent on prescription drugs [31]. This drug budget is increasing worldwide and is forecast to rise by an annual average of 6.1% in the US from 2020 to 2027. A key underlying driver of rising costs is the increase in chronic conditions, related to changes in lifestyle and an aging population [32]. Globally, 33% of adults have multiple long-term diseases, rising to 75% in developed countries. Healthcare costs increase with each condition [33], and with age. Annual US treatment costs for an over-65 patient are five times higher than for under 18 s, and 2.5 times those for people aged 18–64 [34]. The number of over-65 s is set to increase significantly in the next 20 years.

At the same time R&D productivity in the pharma industry has been diminishing for decades. In 2018, R&D returns declined to 1.9%, down from 10.1% in 2010 [35]. Drug discovery is costly (at over $2.8B per marketed drug) [36] and lengthy—it takes an average of 12 years to develop and market a new drug [37]. Even then, as noted above, many drugs benefit only a limited proportion of patients to whom they are prescribed [1].

A secondary driver in the increase in drug spending is the growing emphasis in biopharmaceutical innovation away from small molecule drugs to more complex and expensive biologic drugs including targeted antibodies, cancer vaccines, checkpoint inhibitors, and cell and gene therapies. Since 2014, almost all the net growth in drug spending is accounted for by biologic medicines [38]. In 2017, while biologic drugs represented just 2% of all US prescriptions, they accounted for 37% of net drug spending.

There are good reasons underpinning this switch of emphasis—new biologic approaches have been revolutionary in offering new therapy options and more effective modalities for some extremely difficult to treat conditions, especially in oncology. Use of monoclonal antibodies also overcomes a lot of the issues associated with late-stage failure of small molecule compounds due to off-target effects, toxicity and bioavailability.

There is undoubtedly a subset of patients who will only benefit from these treatments and who should therefore have access to them, but the economics of their use can be challenging for widespread adoption by health systems [39]. High cost is a consistent attribute of biologic drugs, which on average cost $10,000–$30,000 per patient per year. This is particularly true in the US where, unlike Europe, these drugs are regulated differently and have considerable protection with relatively little competition from generic versions, known as 'biosimilars' [40]. While potentially transformational for discrete patient sub-groups, this level of pricing for biologics does not always support their widespread use. This presents a challenge for all parties—payers, providers, patients and even the pharma companies themselves in the longer run. Precision medicine is a key tool in ensuring that medicines are prescribed to those who can benefit from them, saving cost and improve patient treatment.

4.2 Using patient stratification to inform drug repurposing

As of 2018, over 1500 drugs have been approved [41, 42], including many safe and effective medicines that hit targets that play roles in multiple diseases. These can be used in other disease areas with a somewhat lower regulatory burden as they have already been safely prescribed (often for decades) in humans.

Traditionally, drug repurposing involves identifying a drug candidate that is proven safe in humans but that was either ineffective for its original indication, or that has been approved and launched in another disease area. Someone wishing to repurpose the drug would typically license it from the original inventor or company marketing the drug, reformulate it if necessary, and then take it through a shortened clinical trial in the new indication, before gaining approval and launch. This can be quicker and cheaper than *de novo* drug development. Repurposing can help identify therapies especially for areas of unmet medical need in complex disease such as asthma, ALS, dementia and breast cancer [43].

The detailed disease architecture views offered by the combinatorial approach used by **precision**life **MARKERS** take drug repurposing from a serendipitous exercise, observing multiple metabolic roles or potential poly-pharmacology of specific targets, to a level where diseases can be systematic repurposed, identifying all of the available therapies for targets that are relevant to the various disease population sub-groups (**Figure** 7).

4.2.1 Identifying drug repurposing opportunities systematically in breast cancer

Breast cancer is a highly heterogeneous disease with significant variations in prognosis, treatment response across the patient population. It is currently the leading cause of cancer-related mortality in women [44], with approximately 1 in

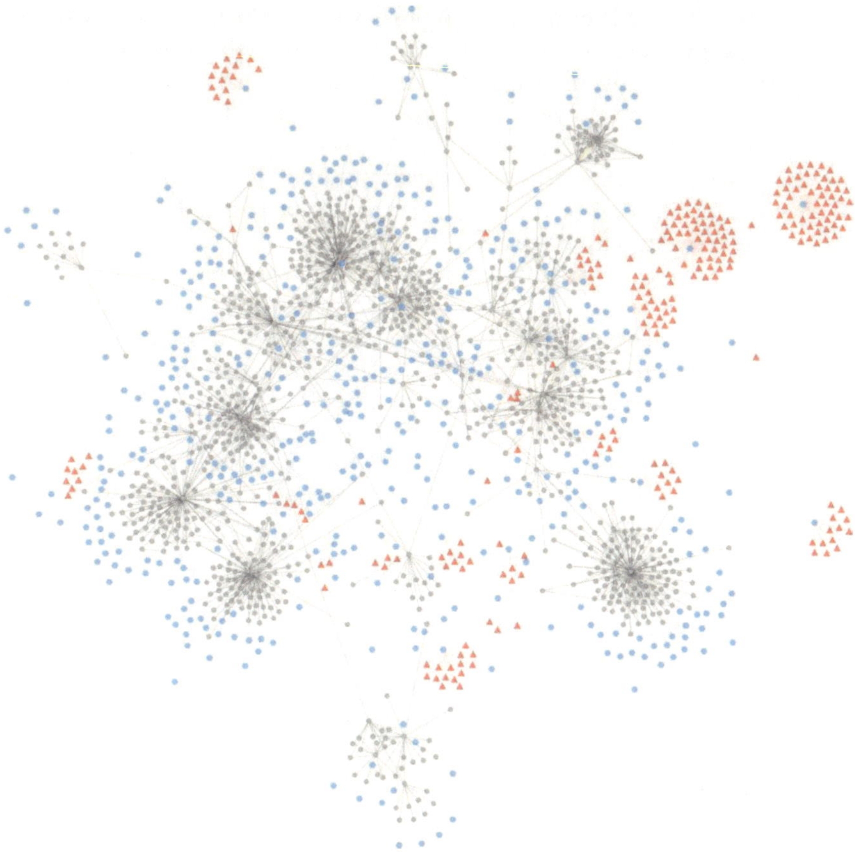

Figure 7.
Detailed disease architecture view of the SNPs (grey circles) and genes (blue circles) associated with ALS disease risk from a ***precisionlife MARKERS*** *study of 8700 patients and 14,400 controls. This connects patient sub-groups with the genes/targets involved in their disease and the available drugs/development compounds known to be active against all of these targets (red triangles).*

8 women being diagnosed with the disease at some point in their lifetime [45]. Patients are currently classified into several different molecular subtypes, based on underlying disease mechanisms, hormone receptor status and tumour biology. Common forms include ER, PR and HER2-positive and triple-negative breast cancer (TNBC).

Some of these have existing targeted therapies. Greater understanding of underlying HER2-positive disease mechanisms has led to the development of HER2-targeted therapies such as trastuzumab and lapatinib, generating significant improvements in patient survival as a result [46]. Notwithstanding these improvements, up to 50% of HER2-positive breast cancer patients still go on to develop metastases.

However, although breast cancer treatment has a more personalized approach than some other diseases, subtypes of breast cancer patients—such as those with TNBC—do not respond to these targeted hormonal therapies. These may correspond to more aggressive and harder to treat forms of the disease. Because of this there remains a significant need for more therapeutic options and greater personalization of treatment strategies in breast cancer therapy in order to continue to increase patient response rates and overall survival.

In order to investigate potential repurposing options for one key sub-group of patients who do not have as many therapeutic options, we wanted to stratify the breast cancer population and run a systematic repurposing study to identify all of the known active chemical compounds. Again, we used the UK Biobank to generate the study population (cases and controls). Unfortunately, the hormone receptor status of the patients is not routinely available in the dataset, so tying these to disease phenotype at a very detailed level was not possible.

Genotype data of 547,197 SNPs from 11,088 breast-cancer cases and 22,176 controls (1:2 case control ratio all women) was obtained from the UK Biobank (ICD10 code C50) [47]. An age-matched control set was created of randomly selected healthy females with no prior history of cancer. We ran the **precision**life **MARKERS** platform to identify disease associated signatures.

The results of the study are a series of SNPs, scored and ranked to select the most significant mutations. These are then mapped to genes and annotated using data from a wide range of publicly available data sources. Information on the functional role, pathways and expression levels for these genes is combined with information on active chemistry, druggability, on- and off-target effects, toxicity, bioavailability, as well as assays, models, scientific literature, IP filings and other sources.

A series of heuristics were then applied on the identified genes to find the targets and candidate drugs with the highest potential for repurposing on the basis of their correlation to disease, their existing disease indications, and other criteria such as expression in relevant (disease-related) tissues, acceptable safety profiles, delivery route, formulations and patent scope.

We found 175 risk-associated genes that are relevant to different patient subpopulations. These genes were annotated and analyzed using the druggability heuristics discussed above. Using *in silico* tests, we identified 23 gene targets as high scoring repurposing candidates.

Different diseases may share common pathways, and drugs that affect genes in these pathways could therefore treat a variety of disease indications. Mapping existing drugs onto the genetic and metabolic signatures (**Figure 8**) indicates areas where there are already good clinical options, and also where off-label use of existing therapeutics with good safety and tolerability profiles, with acceptable routes of administration, could have potential. For a given patient, their specific combination of SNPs will in large part determine which drug or combination of drugs are likely to benefit them personally.

4.2.2 Our methodology identified two existing repurposed breast cancer drugs

Two of the targets we identified in our breast cancer study, *P4HA2* and *TGM2*, which were both identified as having high repurposing potential, have already been investigated in the context of breast cancer and therefore serve as useful validation examples.

One of the highest scored genes identified in the analysis was *P4HA2*, whose protein product plays a role in collagen synthesis, catalyzing the formation of crucial 4-hydroxyproline residues that are involved in collagen helix formation and stabilization [48]. Collagen deposition in breast cancer increases cancer cell development and growth [49]. Inhibiting *P4HA2* may therefore prove beneficial in breast cancer by reducing collagen synthesis and deposition.

Even as well-known and ubiquitous a drug as aspirin decreases the expression of *P4HA2*, and thus lowering collagen deposition [50]. Aspirin is very well-studied [51], with a wealth of pharmacokinetic and toxicology data at high- and low-dose. It has a simple molecular structure (see **Figure 9**), meaning that it is notorious for interacting with a wide variety of biological targets. It was originally licensed as a non-selective COX-2 inhibitor [52], however it also modulates several different transcription factors and pathways implicated in cancer, including NF-κB, PIK3CA and AMPK and mTORC1 signalling [53].

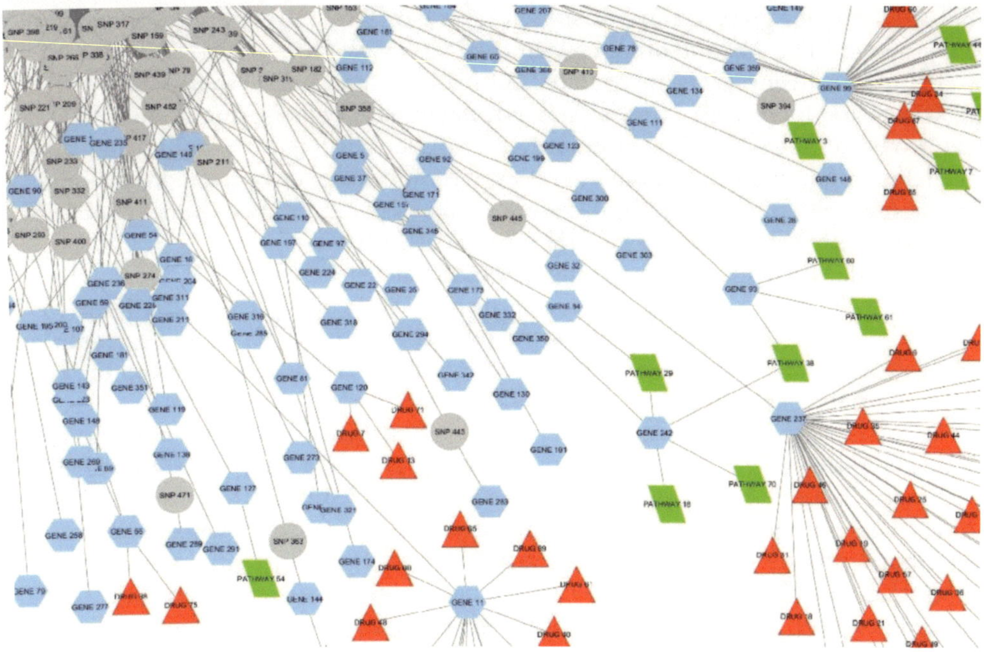

Figure 8.
Graph of existing drug options for key targets identified as being relevant to disease sub-populations in a breast cancer population.

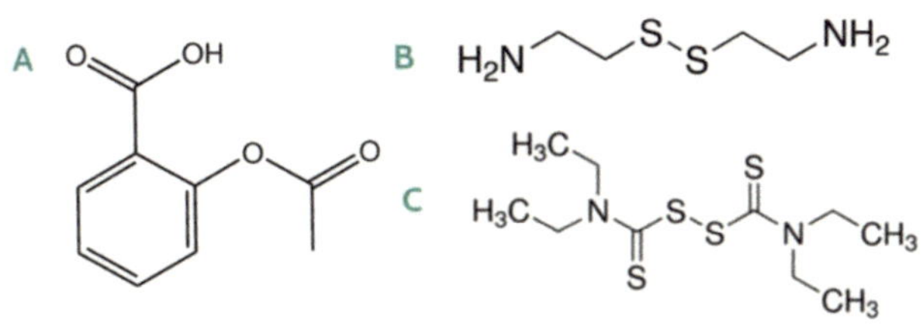

Figure 9.
Molecular structures of aspirin (A), cystamine (B) and disulfiram (C).

Aspirin reduces *P4HA2* activity through two different mechanisms [50] and also enhances the levels of an miRNA called let-7 g, which binds and suppresses the expression of *P4HA2*. Additionally, the promoter of *P4HA2* has three NF-κB binding sites and aspirin inhibits NF-κB expression, resulting in a concomitant decrease in *P4HA2* activity. The benefits of this aspirin-induced reduction in collagen deposition were observed in a model of hepatocellular carcinoma, where inhibition of *P4HA2* resulted in a reduction in tumour growth.

There is however conflicting evidence as to whether aspirin is effective in both reducing the risk of breast cancer and improving disease survival after diagnosis [53, 54]. A greater understanding of the mechanisms behind aspirin's anti-tumour effect and stratification of the population into more clinically relevant subsets may indicate groups of patients who are more likely to respond to aspirin treatment. Our results identified a sub-group of patients with a gene signature that indicates aberrant *P4HA2* expression for whom administration of aspirin is more likely to be effective.

TGM2 also scored highly for repurposing potential. *TGM2* encodes an enzyme (transglutaminase 2, TG2) involved in post-translation modification of proteins, facilitating their crosslinking [55]. High TG2 expression has been associated with increased tumour growth and invasion in several different cancer types through the activation of PI3K/Akt and other cell survival pathways [56].

In breast cancer, TG2 is upregulated compared to its baseline in normal epithelial tissue, and increasing expression is correlated with higher tumour stage [57]. It has also been shown that TG2 interacts with interleukin-6 (IL-6), facilitating IL-6 mediated inflammation, tumour aggressiveness and metastasis in a mouse model of breast cancer [57]. Hence, repurposing a TG2 inhibitor in breast cancer could be therapeutically beneficial in a specific subtype of patients.

Cystamine is an allosteric inhibitor of TG2, causing the formation of a disulfide bond between two cysteine residues, diminishing TG2's catalytic activity [58]. Moreover, although cystamine has not yet been trialled in breast cancer patients, an *in vitro* study has found that inhibiting TG2 expression resulted in reduced breast tumour growth compared to controls [59].

Unfortunately, trials in humans demonstrate that cystamine can cause a range of dose-limiting side effects [60]. Conversely, disulfiram, a drug approved for the treatment of chronic alcoholism, has a comparable molecular structure to cystamine (see **Figure 9**). Palanski et al. demonstrated that disulfiram has the same activity as cystamine *in vitro*, with comparable inhibitory constants when assessed experimentally [61]. Disulfiram has a more favourable pharmacokinetic profile than cystamine; it can be administered orally with a maximum dose of 500 mg/day and is reasonably well tolerated in patients [62, 63].

Both targets identified from this study, *TGM2* and *P4HA2*, have strong mechanistic links to breast cancer and are targeted by approved drugs with favourable pharmacokinetic and toxicity profiles. These two example targets demonstrate the potential of this approach to systematically identify repurposing candidates that have potential to be effective in specific sub-groups of breast cancer patients.

The analysis of multifactorial, multi-omic datasets using **precisionlife MARKERS** identifies disease associated combinations of features, provides an important improvement in analytical capability that will be central to the delivery all aspects of precision medicine. This will enable development of more detailed insights and personalized medicine strategies, with the potential to target specific sub-types of diseases with the greatest unmet need, such as triple negative breast cancer.

5. Combinatorial therapy design

Recognition of the need for more personalized prescription using all available information has driven huge interest in precision medicine, but progress has been slower outside of oncology [64]. The combination of large quantities of patient genotype, phenotype and clinical data and improved data analytics methods have the potential to usher in a new era of affordable precision medicine, lowering the cost of care and identifying the best drugs for individual patients, thereby giving them the best possible outcome. In a time of rising drug costs and squeezes on healthcare budgets, this step could be crucially important for the future affordability of healthcare.

5.1 Personalized therapy selection

Repurposing drugs on an individual patient basis, through off-label prescribing, is already a route that can provide immediate access to effective drugs for patients with unmet needs. It is not without significant problematic issues, but

Drug/Combination	Approved Indication	Off Label Use
Minipress (prazosin)	Hypertension	Post-traumatic stress disorder
Provigil (modafinil)	Sleep disorders	Depression
Statin, metformin (type 2 diabetes), doxycycline (antibiotic) and mebendazole (anti-worming agent)		Glioblastoma

Table 1.
Examples of current common off-label prescriptions.

off-label prescribing already accounts for 20% of US out-patient prescriptions [65]. Including the examples shown below (**Table 1**) [66, 67].

More widespread delivery of precision medicine in the future could be achieved by having a principled and evidence led basis from which to make personalized suggestions for an individual patient, and then studying the outcomes for patients and using these to refine future prescriptions [68]. This would need to be confirmed with appropriate biomarker tests (such as the combinatorial disease signatures described above) and subject to review as part of a personalized health plan by a comprehensive clinical team as is the current practice in oncology precision medicine applications [69].

Payers and prescribers routinely collect such data over a sufficiently long time, and with appropriate controls, this can be used to identify a patient as a responder or non-responder to a particular treatment. Given the N-of-1 nature of the trials, the recommendations may also include off-label prescriptions, potentially including the full range of drugs available on the formulary, including generics. Recent studies have shown the efficacy and therapeutic benefits of choosing such non-standard drug options when guided by genomic insights, especially in diseases such as colon cancer [70, 71]. When available these may reduce the dosage of high toxic chemotherapy agents required while providing more targeted therapies that increase the effectiveness of treatment.

The key to maintaining effective oversight and control of such personalized interventions and deriving full benefit from them for future public health will be dependent on harmonizing their design and collection of their results. Aggregated results of many N-of-1 trials (with harmonized design and data capture) will offer an on-going information resource that can be used to identify how to better treat subsets of the population or even the population at large [1].

In the future, payers and prescribers will be able to use a clinical decision support tool based on the insights from a detailed combinatorial analysis of the disease architecture plus the results of the N-of-1 real world trials to prescribe existing drugs, either as approved or off-label, on a personalized basis to individual patients (see **Figure 10**). The additional therapeutic options from systematic repurposing, coupled with use of coordinated clinical decision support tools and structured N-of-1 trials will be designed to optimize the prescription of effective drugs, single or in combinations. This process could speed up the process of effective treatment for both the patient and the physician, cut costs, improve outcomes, and reduce side-effects.

Adding further datasets, such as known drug:drug, drug:disease and even drug:food interactions, and feeding back patient/clinician reported outcomes will further improve the personalization of recommendations for the patient, enabling the avoidance of predictable side-effects and adverse drug reaction with a patient's other medications. It also present new opportunities to involve them as an active partner in the management of their own health, for example by providing personalized dietary advice that minimizes predictable adverse drug reactions [72].

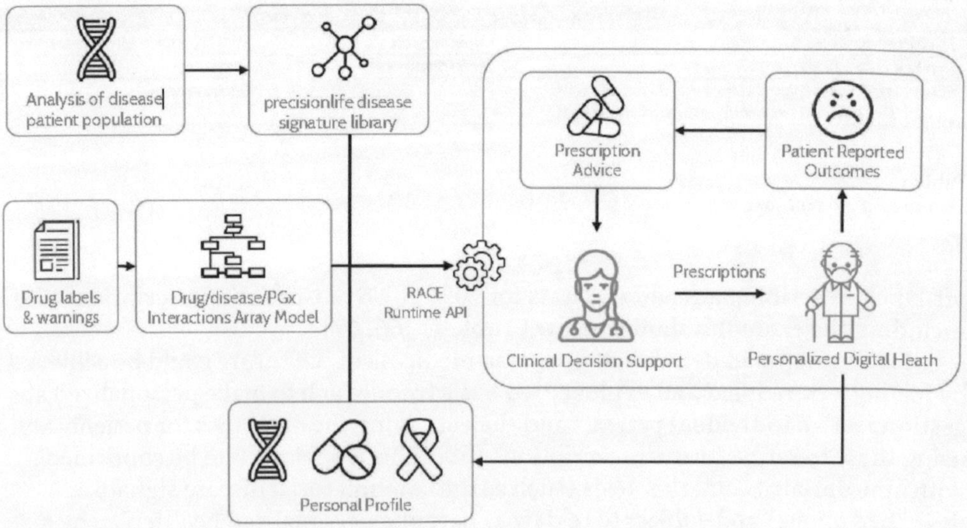

Figure 10.
Overview of clinical decision support system providing personalized therapy selection and patient lifestyle/diet advisory tools alongside a learning framework build on patient reported outcomes.

6. Conclusions

Datasets are now being compiled in routine healthcare that give an unprecedentedly detailed and holistic view of patients. New AI and analytical tools are beginning to combine and analyze these data to improve diagnosis and the development and selection of therapies that are more closely targeted at specific patient sub-groups. These create opportunities to transform the delivery of medicine in the near future.

The combination of better access large quantities of high-quality multi-omic patient data, improved data analytics, systematic drug repurposing and N-of-1 trials have the potential to usher in a new era of affordable, personalized and precision medicine. This could lower the cost of care and identify the best drugs for individual patients, thereby giving them the best outcomes possible. In a time of rising drug costs and squeezes on healthcare budgets, this step could be crucially important for the future of healthcare.

The insights generated by multifactorial and multi-omic analysis of large disease populations are particularly enabling to:

- accelerate innovative drug discovery and repurposing projects
- find novel validated and stratified targets for complex diseases
- identify multi-omic biomarkers for patient stratification
- build better, more personalized combinatorial risk scores
- inform clinical decision support systems for precision medicine

Acknowledgements

Some of this work has been conducted using the UK Biobank Resource, which has provided high quality patient datasets for a variety of disease studies. Special thanks to Gert Møller and the rest of the PrecisionLife team, who developed some of the novel analytical technologies discussed.

Author details

Steve Gardner*, Sayoni Das and Krystyna Taylor
PrecisionLife Ltd., Oxon, UK

*Address all correspondence to: steve@precisionlife.com

References

[1] Schork NJ. Personalized medicine: Time for one-person trials. Nature. 2015;**520**(7549):609-611. DOI: 10.1038/520609a

[2] Currie GP, Lee DKC, Lipworth BJ. Long-acting β2-agonists in asthma. Drug Safety. 2006;**29**:647-656

[3] Ginsburg GS, McCarthy JJ. Personalized medicine: Revolutionizing drug discovery and patient care. TIBS. 2001;**19**:491-496

[4] Greenberg PE, Fournier AA, Sisitsky T, Pike CT, Kessler RC. The economic burden of adults with major depressive disorder in the United States (2005 and 2010). The Journal of Clinical Psychiatry. 2015;**76**:155-162

[5] Staff Writer. UnitedHealthcare to Cover Genetic Testing for Precision Medicine in Depression, Anxiety. Clinical OMICs. 2 August 2019. Available from: https://www.clinicalomics.com/topics/molecular-dx-topic/unitedhealthcare-to-cover-genetic-testing-for-precision-medicine-in-depression-anxiety/

[6] Tam V, Patel N, Turcotte M, Bossé Y, Paré G, Meyre D. Benefits and limitations of genome-wide association studies. Nature Reviews Genetics. 2019;**20**:467-484. DOI: 10.1038/s41576-019-0127-1

[7] Boyle EA, Li YI, Pritchard JK. An expanded view of complex traits: From polygenic to Omnigenic. Cell. 2017;**169**:1177-1186

[8] Morgan P et al. Impact of a five-dimensional framework on R&D productivity at AstraZeneca. Nature Reviews Drug Discovery. 2018;**17**:167-181

[9] Nelson MR et al. The support of human genetic evidence for approved drug indications at GSK. Nature Genetics. 2015;**47**:856-862

[10] King EA, Davis JW, Degner JF. Revised estimates of the impact of genetic support for drug mechanisms on drug approvals. PLOS Genetics. 2019;**15**(12):e1008489. DOI: 10.1371/journal.pgen.1008489

[11] Fruman DA, Chiu H, Hopkins BD, Bagrodia S, Cantley LC, Abraham RT. The PI3K pathway in human disease. Cell. 2017;**170**:605-635

[12] Wong K-K, Engelman JA, Cantley LC. Targeting the PI3K signaling pathway in cancer. Current Opinion in Genetics & Development. 2010;**20**:87. DOI: 10.1016/j.gde.2009.11.002

[13] Mellerup E, Andreassen OA, Bennike B, Dam H, Djurovic S, Jorgensen MB, et al. Combinations of genetic variants associated with bipolar disorder. PLOS One. 2017;**12**(12):e0189739. DOI: 10.1371/journal.pone.0189739

[14] Ahlqvist E et al. Novel subgroups of adult-onset diabetes and their association with outcomes: A data-driven cluster analysis of six variables. The Lancet Diabetes and Endocrinology. 2018;**6**:361-369. DOI: 10.1016/S2213-8587(18)30051-2

[15] Sudlow C et al. UK biobank: An open access resource for identifying the causes of a wide range of complex diseases of middle and old age. PLOS Medicine. 2015;**12**(3):e1001779. DOI: 10.1371/journal.pmed.1001779

[16] Van Rheenen W, Pulit SL, Dekker AM, et al. Project MinE: Study design and pilot analyses of a large-scale whole-genome sequencing study in amyotrophic lateral sclerosis. European Journal of Human Genetics.

2018;**26**:1537-1546. DOI: 10.1038/s41431-018-0177-4

[17] Asthma UK. Available from: https://www.asthma.org.uk/about/media/facts-and-statistics [Accessed: 13 August 2019]

[18] Baos S, Calzada D, Cremades-Jimeno L, et al. Nonallergic asthma and its severity: Biomarkers for its discrimination in peripheral samples. Frontiers in Immunology. 2018;**9**:1416

[19] Kim KW, Ober C. Lessons learned from GWAS of asthma. Allergy, Asthma & Immunology Research. 2019;**11**(2):170-187

[20] Ferreira MAR, Mathur R, Vonk JM, et al. Genetic architectures of childhood- and adult-onset asthma are partly distinct. American Journal of Human Genetics. 2019;**104**(4):665-684

[21] Carr TF, Zeki AA, Kraft M. Eosinophilic and noneosinophilic asthma. American Journal of Respiratory and Critical Care Medicine. 2018;**197**(1):22-37

[22] Lee JY, Zhao L, Youn HS, et al. Saturated fatty acid activates but polyunsaturated fatty acid inhibits toll-like receptor 2 dimerized with toll-like receptor 6 or 1. The Journal of Biological Chemistry. 2004;**279**:16971-16979

[23] Al-Khami AA, Ghonim MA, Del Valle L, et al. Fuelling the mechanisms of asthma: Increased fatty acid oxidation in inflammatory immune cells may represent a novel therapeutic target. Clinical and Experimental Allergy. 2017;**47**(9):1170-1184

[24] Sedgwick JB, Hwang YS, Gerbyshak HA, et al. Oxidized low-density lipoprotein activates migration and degranulation of human granulocytes. American Journal of Respiratory Cell and Molecular Biology. 2003;**29**(6):702-709

[25] Alvarnas JC. "Healthcare Perspective" Oncology in the Precision Medicine Era. Cham: Springer; 2020. pp. 1-12

[26] Davis JC, Furstenthal L, Desai AA, Norris T, Sutaria S, Fleming E, et al. The microeconomics of personalized medicine: Today's challenge and tomorrow's promise. Nature Reviews. Drug Discovery. 2009;**8**(4):279-286

[27] Personalized Medicine Coalition. The Personalized Medicine Report 2017. 2017. Available from: http://www.personalizedmedicinecoalition.org/Userfiles/PMC-Corporate/file/The-Personalized-Medicine-Report1.pdf

[28] CMS.gov. National Health Expenditure Data: Historical. 2019. Available from: https://www.cms.gov/research-statistics-data-and-systems/statistics-trends-and-reports/nationalhealthexpenddata/nationalhealthaccountshistorical.html

[29] Office of the Actuary at the Centers for Medicare & Medicaid Services (CMS). National Health Expenditure Projections, 2018-2027: Economic and Demographic Trends Drive Spending and Enrollment Growth. Baltimore, MD, USA: Centers for Medicare and Medicaid Services; 2019. DOI: 10.1377/hlthaff.2018.05499

[30] EFPIA. The Pharma Industry in Figures—Economy: With a Focus on World Pharmaceutical Market. European Federation of Pharmaceutical Industries and Associations. 2017. Available from: https://www.efpia.eu/publications/data-center/the-pharma-industry-in-figures-economy/world-pharmaceutical-market [Accessed: 27 June 2019]

[31] CMS.gov. Nation's Health Dollar—Where It Came from, Where It Went. 2019. Available from: https://www.cms.gov/Research-Statistics-Data-and-Systems/Statistics-Trends-and-Reports/NationalHealthExpendData/Downloads/PieChartSourcesExpenditures.pdf

[32] CMS.gov. National Health Expenditure Projections 2018-2027. 2019. Available from: https://www.cms.gov/Research-Statistics-Data-and-Systems/Statistics-Trends-and-Reports/NationalHealthExpendData/Downloads/ForecastSummary.pdf

[33] Hajat C, Stein E. The global burden of multiple chronic conditions: A narrative review. Preventive Medical Reports. 2018;**12**:284-293. DOI: 10.1016/j.pmedr.2018.10.008

[34] AHRQ. Medical Expenditure Panel Survey. 2017. Available from: https://meps.ahrq.gov/mepstrends/hc_use/

[35] Deloitte Centre for Health Solutions. Unlocking R&D Productivity: Measuring the Return from Pharmaceutical Innovation 2018. 2018. Available from https://www2.deloitte.com/content/dam/Deloitte/uk/Documents/life-sciences-health-care/deloitte-uk-measuring-return-on-pharma-innovation-report-2018.pdf

[36] Policy & Medicine. A Tough Road: Cost to Develop One New Drug is $2.6 billion; Approval Rate for Drugs Entering Clinical Development is Less Than 12%. Available from: https://www.policymed.com/2014/12/a-tough-road-cost-to-develop-one-new-drug-is-26-billion-approval-rate-for-drugs-entering-clinical-de.html [Accessed: 28 November 2019]

[37] Van N, Drugs GA. Devices, and the FDA: Part 1: An overview of approval processes for Drugs. JACC: Basic to Translational Science. 2016;**1**(3):170-179

[38] IQVIA Institute Report. Medicine Use and Spending in the US. 2018. Available from: https://www.iqvia.com/institute/reports/medicine-use-and-spending-in-the-us-review-of-2017-outlook-to-2022

[39] Chen BK, Yang YT, Bennett CL. Why biologics and biosimilars remain so expensive. Drugs. 2018;**78**:1777-1781

[40] Tribble SJ. Why the U.S. Remains the World's Most Expensive Market for 'Biologic' Drugs. Kaiser Health News; 2018. Available from: https://khn.org/news/u-s-market-for-biologic-drugs-is-most-expensive-in-the-world/

[41] Kinch MS, Haynesworth A, Kinch SL, Hoyer D. An overview of FDA-approved new molecular entities: 1827-2013. Drug Discovery Today. 2014;**19**(8):1033-1039

[42] Mullard A. 2018 FDA drug approvals. Nature Reviews. Drug Discovery. 2019;**18**(2):85-89

[43] Nosengo N. Can you teach old drugs new tricks? Nature. 2016;**534**: 314-316

[44] World Health Organisation. Breast Cancer. 2019. Available from: https://www.who.int/cancer/prevention/diagnosis-screening/breast-cancer/en/ [Accessed: 28 November 2019]

[45] NHS. 'One in Eight' Will Get Breast Cancer. 2011. Available from: https://www.nhs.uk/news/cancer/one-in-eight-will-get-breast-cancer/ [Accessed: 28 November 2019]

[46] Pernas S, Tolaney SM. HER2-positive breast cancer: New therapeutic frontiers and overcoming resistance. Therapeutic Advances in Medical Oncology. 2019;**11**:1758835919833519

[47] Bycroft C, Freeman C, Petkova D, Band G, Elliott LT, Sharp K, et al. The UK Biobank resource with deep phenotyping and genomic data. Nature. 2018;**562**(7726):203-209

[48] Xiong G, Stewart RL, Chen J, Gao T, Scott TL, Samayoa LM, et al. Collagen prolyl 4-hydroxylase 1 is essential for HIF-1α stabilization and TNBC chemoresistance. Nature Communications. 2018;**9**(1):4456

[49] Xiong G, Deng L, Zhu J, Rychahou PG, Xu R. Prolyl-4-hydroxylase α

subunit 2 promotes breast cancer progression and metastasis by regulating collagen deposition. BMC Cancer. 2014;**14**:1

[50] Wang T, Fu X, Jin T, Zhang L, Liu B, Wu Y, et al. Aspirin targets P4HA2 through inhibiting NFκB and LMCD1-AS1/let-7g to inhibit tumour growth and collagen deposition in hepatocellular carcinoma. eBioMedicine. 2019;**45**:168-180

[51] Goldberg DR. Aspirin: Turn-of-the-Century Miracle Drug. Science History Institute; 2009. Available from: https://www.sciencehistory.org/distillations/magazine/aspirin-turn-of-the-century-miracle-drug [Accessed: 29 November 2019]

[52] Henry WS, Laszewski T, Tsang T, Beca F, Beck AH, McAllister SS, et al. Aspirin suppresses growth in PI3K-mutant breast cancer by activating AMPK and inhibiting mTORC1 Signaling. Cancer Research. 2017;77(3):790-801

[53] Frisk G, Ekberg S, Lidbrink E, Eloranta S, Sund M, Fredriksson I, et al. No association between low-dose aspirin use and breast cancer outcomes overall: A Swedish population-based study. Breast Cancer Research. 2018;**20**:142

[54] Elwood PC, Pickering JE, Morgan G, Galante J, Weightman AL, Morris D, et al. Systematic review update of observational studies further supports aspirin role in cancer treatment: Time to share evidence and decision-making with patients? PLOS One. 2018;**13**(9):e0203957

[55] Tatsukawa H, Furutani Y, Hitomi K, Kojima S. Transglutaminase 2 has opposing roles in the regulation of cellular functions as well as cell growth and death. Cell Death & Disease. 2016;7(6):e2244

[56] Szondy Z, Korponay-Szabó I, Király R, Sarang Z, Tsay GJ. Transglutaminase 2 in human diseases. Biomedicine (Taipei). 2017;7(3):15

[57] Oh K, Ko E, Kim HS, Park AK, Moon HG, Noh DY, et al. Transglutaminase 2 facilitates the distant hematogenous metastasis of breast cancer by modulating interleukin-6 in cancer cells. Breast Cancer Research. 2011;**13**(5):R96

[58] Stamnaes J, Pinkas DM, Fleckenstein B, Khosla C, Sollid LM. Redox regulation of transglutaminase 2 activity. The Journal of Biological Chemistry. 2010;**285**(33):25402-25409

[59] Oh K, Lee O, Park Y, Won Seo M, Lee DS. IL-1β induces IL-6 production and increases invasiveness and estrogen-independent growth in a TG2-dependent manner in human breast cancer cells. BMC Cancer. 2016;**16**:724

[60] Dubinsky R, Gray C. CYTE-I-HD: Phase I dose finding and tolerability study of cysteamine (Cystagon) in Huntington's disease. Movement Disorders. 2005;**21**(4):530-533

[61] Palanski BA, Khosla C. Cystamine and Disulfiram inhibit human transglutaminase 2 via an oxidative mechanism. Biochemistry. 2018;**57**(24):3359-3363

[62] Mutschler J, Dirican G, Gutzeit A, Grosshans M. Safety and efficacy of long-term disulfiram aftercare. Clinical Neuropharmacology. 2011;**34**(5):195-198

[63] National Institute for Health and Care Excellence (NICE). Disulfiram. 2019. Available from: https://bnf.nice.org.uk/drug/disulfiram.html [Accessed: 29 November 2019]

[64] Pushpakom S et al. Drug repurposing: Progress, challenges and recommendations. Nature Reviews. Drug Discovery. 2019;**18**:41-58

[65] AHRQ. Off-Label Drugs: What You Need to Know. 2015. Available from: https://www.webmd.com/a-to-z-guides/features/off-label-drug-use-what-you-need-to-know#1.

[66] O'Shea T. 10 Surprising Off-Label Uses for Prescription Medications. Pharmacy Times; 2016. Available from: https://www.pharmacytimes.com/contributor/timothy-o-shea/2016/01/10-surprising-off-label-uses-for-prescription-medications

[67] Staff Writer. "Repurposing" Off-Patent Drugs Offers Big Hopes of New Treatments. The Economist; 2019. Available from: https://www.economist.com/international/2019/02/28/repurposing-off-patent-drugs-offers-big-hopes-of-new-treatments

[68] Ginsburg SG, Phillips KA. Precision medicine: From science to value. Health Affairs (Millwood). 2018;**37**:694-701

[69] Thompson MA, Godden JJ, Weissman SM, Wham D, Wilson A, Ruggeri A, et al. Implementing an oncology precision medicine clinic in a large community health system. The American Journal of Managed Care. August 2017;**23**(10 Spec No.):SP425-SP427

[70] Bangi E, Murgia C, Teague AG, Sansom OJ, Cagan RL. Functional exploration of colorectal cancer genomes using drosophila. Nature Communications. 2016;**29**:13615. DOI: 10.1038/ncomms13615

[71] Wilson C. Specially Created Animal 'Cancer Avatars' Could Personalise Treatments. New Scientist; 2019. Available from: https://www.newscientist.com/article/2204384-specially-created-animal-cancer-avatars-could-personalise-treatments/

[72] Gardner SP, Pawlowski M, Møller GL, Jensen CE. Delivering personalized dietary advice for health management and disease prevention. Digital Medicine. 2018;**4**:127-132. DOI: 10.4103/digm.digm_19_18

Section 4

Patient Perspectives

Chapter 8

Toward the Clinic: Understanding Patient Perspectives on AI and Data-Sharing for AI-Driven Oncology Drug Development

Roberta Dousa

Abstract

The increasing application of AI-led systems for oncology drug development and patient care holds the potential to usher pronounced impacts for patients' well-being. Beyond technical innovations and infrastructural adjustments, research suggests that realizing this potential also hinges upon patients' trust and understanding. With the promise of precision oncology predicated on a data-driven approach, public and private survey studies indicate patients view the lack of clarity surrounding data privacy, security, and ownership as a growing concern. Assuming an in-depth, semi-structured interview protocol, this qualitative study examines cancer patients' perceptions of the burgeoning development of AI-led systems for oncology as well as their perspectives on sharing health data (including genetic data) for drug development. This article seeks to provide greater insight into the legal and ethical challenges that surround the application of these tools and to explore patient-centered approaches to building the frameworks of trust and accountability crucial to transferring these advances to the clinic.

Keywords: AI, oncology drug development, health data-sharing, cancer patients

1. Introduction

Recent decades have witnessed major advances for AI systems, which has subsequently resulted in increased interest in applying AI-driven technologies for oncology drug development and cancer patient care. Beyond technical and infrastructural adjustments, improvements, and innovations, recent studies suggest that realizing the potential of AI in healthcare and applying data-driven models to oncology drug development hinges in part upon the public's—with especial regard to potential patients' and users'—trust and understanding. As contingent to oncology drug development and research, the importance of the public's capacity for trust extends to both the use of AI and data-sharing. Public and private survey studies indicate patients view the lack of clarity surrounding data privacy, security, and ownership as a growing concern. Exemplifying this, in September 2018, a KPMG survey of over 2000 Britons found that 51% of its participants were both worried about data privacy and unwilling to share personal data with U.K. organizations for AI research and use [1]. In addition, the U.K.'s Academic Health Sciences

IntechOpen

Network, in conjunction with the Department of Health and Social Care, released a report delineating the results from a 2018 "state of the nation survey." Similar to the findings of the KPMG survey, this report, titled "Accelerating Artificial Intelligence in Health and Care," identified that, according to pioneers in the field, the "overall enablers" to realizing the potential of AI in health and care include an 'ethical framework to build/preserve trust and transparency' as well as "clarity around ownership of data" [2]. Likewise, when asked, "which of the following areas do you think will be the greatest problem for artificial intelligence," the KPMG survey respondents' top answer was "data privacy and security."

As patients increasingly view the lack of clarity surrounding data privacy, security, and ownership as a growing concern, the potential benefits of AI-led oncology drug development and oncology care systems must not be accepted as superseding their potential to enact social harm. As public and patient approval and participation contribute to the use and development of these systems is imperative to study patient perceptions of AI and AI-led oncology drug development endeavors and to heed and address public concerns. Accordingly, this chapter enlists and examines ethnographic, textual, and other qualitative data that the author has assembled in pursuing a broad examination of the legal, political, and ethical imperatives surrounding the development of AI-driven systems for healthcare and for oncology, specifically. This chapter provides new evidence for understanding patient reception of the development and deployment of these systems as well as patients' perceptions and willingness to participate in health-related AI development by sharing medical data, necessary to build these systems and advance their efficacy, with the public and private entities engaged in developing them. Rooted firmly in interview work produced utilizing an in-depth, semi-structured interview protocol this chapter offers insights into the legal and ethical quandaries that surround the application of these tools in order to ultimately explore and assess patient-centered approaches to building crucial frameworks of trust and accountability fundamental to transferring these advances into clinical settings for the betterment of patient outcomes.

This chapter opens by offering a contextual scaffolding to understanding the terms AI and machine learning. Subsequently, the author provides an introductory overview to understand how AI-led systems might be applied to clinical contexts and oncology setting, respectively. This is followed by a discussion of some practical considerations and challenges to AI-enabled healthcare applications. The author then provides an overview of the study's methods and methodology to further contextualize the remaining discussion, which relies heavily upon the author's original qualitative research. This leads to a discussion of patient perceptions, knowledge, and concerns regarding AI-driven systems for oncology, drug development, and medicine, more broadly. Immediately after, the author stages an exploration of patient perceptions and concerns regarding sharing their medical data to bolster AI and oncology drug development research. The final section of this chapter discusses further patient-centered recommendations and proposals for ensuring patient trust, participation, and safety pertinent to increasing the development and clinical use of AI systems for oncology.

2. Defining AI and machine learning

2.1 Defining AI systems and intelligence

Although conceptions of sentient, machinic animacies can be traced as far back as antiquity, the understanding of "AI" or "artificial intelligence" as a term and field of study originated in 1956 following a conference organized at Dartmouth College by the American computer scientist, John McCarthy. McCarthy, who himself coined the term, is often hailed as a preeminent pioneer of AI McCarthy defined artificial intelligence as "the science and engineering of intelligent machines" [3]. The ensuing decades saw the salad days of what the analytic philosopher John Haugeland names as "Good Old Fashioned AI" (GOFAI). Within the paradigm GOFAI, artificial intelligence essentially referred to "procedural, logic-based reasoning and the capacity to manipulate abstract symbolic representations" [4]. For instance, the commercial "expert systems" of the 1970s and 1980s are typically understood as exemplifying GOFAI. By 1969, however, data scientists began to seriously question the general viability of AI as well as the initial, florid promise that surrounded these systems. The deflation of these experts, coupled with considerable decreases in grant support and research output, led to an "AI winter," which lasted approximately for the next 20 years until a renewed interest in machine learning techniques propelled AI research forward [5].

In contrast to GOFAI, the "intelligence" at stake in contemporary AI systems is typically understood to imbricate machine learning techniques. Intelligence, in the current paradigm, is thought to derive from systems' abilities to detect patterns across vast datasets and predict outcomes based on probability statistics. In other words, today algorithmic systems are deemed AI provided they process and analyze vast amounts of data, beyond the scope of an individual human, in order to predict and automate certain activities. Critical to understanding AI's consequences for epistemology and social practice, anthropologist of technology M.C. Elish stresses that "the datasets and models used in these systems are not objective representations of reality" as systems that utilize machine learning techniques "can only be thought to 'know' something in the sense that it can correlate certain relevant variables accurately" [4].

With some cognizance of the shifting valences the term accrued in decades since the 1950s, AI might be otherwise understood as "a characteristic or set of capabilities exhibited by a computer that resembles intelligent behavior" although, evidently, delimiting what might be understood as "intelligence" remains a crucial although unresolved and contested dimension in defining AI [6]. Some researchers consider artificial intelligence to be contingent on behavioral demarcations, ostensible when a "computer can sense and act appropriately in a dynamic environment" [6]. Others link intelligence to symbolic processing, exhibited, for instance, when a system can recognize and respond appropriately to speech [6].

2.2 Machine learning: "imposing a shape on data"

Given the breadth of the term's inherent contestations, evolutions, and stubborn fluidity, social researchers of technology such as Tim Hwang and M.C. Elish contend that definitions of artificial intelligence and intelligent systems might be appropriately understood as "moving targets." Rather than possessing a static set of demarcations signaling intelligence, artificially intelligent systems are defined in relation to "existing beliefs, attitudes, and technology" [6]. They argue that the rhetorical power of "artificial intelligence" is found in its "slipperiness": seemingly everyone has an idea of what AI is, and yet everyone's notion is different [6]. In consequence, data scientists and engineers today tend to shy away from the term "artificial intelligence." Indeed, the equivocality of "artificial intelligence" has siloed "AI" as a marketing term rather than a technical one [4].

Current research in artificial intelligence occurs primarily in the field of machine learning (ML). Although "machine learning" was coined in 1959, significant interest in these techniques did not follow until the 1980s following further developments in techniques such as neural networks. Digital medicine researcher, Eric Topol argues that machine learning can be understood as "computers' ability to learn without being explicitly programmed, with more than 50 different approaches like Random Forest, Bayesian networks, Support Vector machine uses"; they are "computer algorithms [that] learn from examples and experiences (datasets) rather than predefined, hard rules-based methods" [5]. Computer scientist Tom Mitchell has elaborated what that "learning" in the context of ML systems refers to. Mitchell writes: "A computer program is said to learn from experience E with respect to some class of tasks T and performance measure P if its performance at tasks in T, as measured by P, improves with experience E" [7].

Put differently, media and communications scholar Taina Bucher explains that although "algorithms are 'trained' on a corpus of data from which they may 'learn' to make certain kinds of decisions without human oversight...machines do not learn in the same sense that humans do." Rather, Bucher argues, "the kind of learning machines do should be understood in a more *functional* sense" [8]. Citing legal scholar Harry Surden, Bucher explains that machine learning-driven systems are "capable of changing their behavior to enhance their performance on some task through experience" [8].

Machine learning is largely enabled by "proliferating data from which models may learn." It follows that enormous datasets are paramount for developing effective ML systems. Machine learning techniques such as logistic regression models, k-nearest neighbors, and neural networks generally "pivot around ways of transforming, constructing, or imposing some kind of shape on the data and using that shape to discover, decide, classify, rank, cluster, recommend, label, or predict what is happening or what will happen" [9]. Bucher underscores that what determines whether to use one technique over another "depends upon the domain (i.e., loan default prediction vs. image recognition), its demonstrated accuracy in classification, and available computational resources, among other concerns" [8].

Machine learning systems are distinct from deterministic algorithms in that "given a particular input, a deterministic algorithm will always produce the same output by passing through the same sequence of steps" while an ML algorithmic system "will learn to predict outputs based on previous examples of relationships between input data and outputs" [8]. In other words, Bucher notes that "in contrast to the strict logical rules of traditional programming, machine learning is about writing programs that learn to solve problems by examples...using data to make models that have certain features" [8]. Feature engineering involves "extracting and selecting the most important aspects of machine learning" [8]. Signaling the constructed subjectivity of the knowledge produced by systems utilizing machine learning techniques, Bucher explains that "the understanding of data and what it represents, then, is not merely the matter of a machine that learns but also of humans who specify the states and outcomes in which they are interested in the first place" [8].

3. AI systems for oncology and oncology drug development

3.1 AI-enabled medical care

AI systems have been deployed in healthcare contexts since at least the 1970s following the development of computer-assisted clinical decision support tools, however the last decade is particularly thought to have been a watershed moment for the nexus of AI systems and healthcare. The advent of so-called big data analytics coupled with crucial advances in machine learning techniques (specifically, the exponential development of new deep learning algorithms), has propelled both the development of, and a far-reaching rejuvenated interest in, applying these models for medical usage. This has compelled technologists, medical researchers, venture capitalists, and media pundits, among others, to question whether the contemporary is witnessing the dawning of a new era of medicine. In the past several years alone, leading-edge advances in machine learning have enabled AI-driven systems to accurately identify heart rhythm abnormalities, predict suicides at a better rate than mental health professionals; to successfully interpret pathology slides of potential neoplastic tissues or medical scans with the same rate of accuracy (at times, even exceeding the rate of accuracy) of that of senior pathologists and radiologists; and to accurately diagnosis both a multitude of eye ailments such as diabetic retinopathy as well as some skin cancers at a similar rate to (and in some instances, better than) medical professionals [5]. Beyond these examples, other current efforts are directed at training AI systems to identify modifications in drug treatment protocols and to predict clinical outcomes.

3.2 AI-enabled cancer care

These celebrated developments, as well as a host of others, have led researchers in oncology-related fields to question how AI systems might be deployed to improve clinical outcomes for patients with cancer. Health researchers are emboldened by the promise that any piece of medical data able to be translated analytically such as "patterns, predictable outcomes, or pair associations" can be effectively evaluated by machines [10]. Currently, AI-based approaches to clinical trial design, pathology, and radiology are being studied for effectiveness with encouraging results. Under development are other promising applications of AI For example, data and medical scientists are endeavoring to integrate and analyze individuals' multi-omics data (such as individuals' genomes) using AI The ultimate goal of this cooperative research is to usher in a new standard of tailored or personalized medical care with the potential to improve clinical outcomes for patients with cancer. While some researchers and data scientists are pursuing the deployment of multi-omics data to improve early diagnosis in oncology, others are hoping AI-enabled approaches will aid in the continuing discovery of new and increasingly sensitive biomarkers for cancer care [10]. Healthcare professionals, researchers, and data scientists hope that, in the near future, complex biomarkers will constitute an improved basis for cancer prevention and diagnosis, offering patients the most optimal treatments based on the particular characteristics of their cancer, and aid medical professionals in determining the likelihood of recurrence [11].

4. Practical considerations and challenges to AI-enabled healthcare

4.1 Contextualizing the hype: AI limitations

Accompanying the renewed interest in applying machine learning techniques to health data has been a buzz of exaggerated claims and overdrawn expectations regarding how quickly and comprehensively AI will transform modern medicine. Digital medicine researcher Eric Topol offers a partial list of the "outlandish expectations" escorting the development AI-enabled healthcare. Some envision that soon these systems will "outperform doctors at all tasks; diagnose the undiagnosable; treat the untreatable; see the unseeable on scans and slides; predict the unpredictable; classify the unclassifiable; eliminate workflow inefficiencies; eliminate hospital admissions and readmissions; eliminate the surfeit of unnecessary jobs; result in 100% medical adherence; produce zero patient harm; and cure cancer" [5]. Instead, Topol and other medical researchers assume a more modest view: AI-driven systems will not serve as a panacea to all the aforementioned predicaments in modern healthcare but will instead gradually serve as an increasingly important tool in addressing these and other issues. Moreover, medical experts and technologists alike contend that the encouraging results AI-driven systems have garnered in fields like pathology and radiology, for example, should be taken neither as a justification for the outsourcing of pathologists and radiologists, nor point to the burgeoning obsolescence of medical specialists as a whole [10]. Rather, they stress that these initial successes should be understood as an "indication that their workload could be optimized and, importantly, the waiting time for patients to receive a diagnosis can be reduced" [10]. In this perspective, over time, the widespread adoption of AI systems in healthcare will result in a crucial leveling of the "medical knowledge landscape" [5]. As a consequence, some medical researchers believe that advances in AI and the eventual adoption of these systems within the realm of healthcare will herald unprecedented advantages to modern medical specialists by "restoring the gift of time" to health professionals allowing them to devote more clinical attention, emotional support, and guidance to patients [5].

4.2 Tempering visions of imminent medical revolutions

While in the past decade, the development of AI systems for use in the medical field has certainly progressed and led to feats that have garnered significant attention, these successes remain arguably limited and the progression of these systems decidedly gradual. Taking the field of narrow AI diagnostics as an example, recent systems have accurately diagnosed skin lesions and pathology slides in the realm of oncology. In cardiology, AI diagnostic systems have accurately interpreted echocardiographic images and electrocardiograms in diagnosing heart abnormalities [5]. Other AI diagnostic systems have successfully analyzed audio-wave forms to assist in diagnosing asthma, pneumonia, tuberculosis, and other lung ailments [5]. All of these successes, however, constitute narrow AI tools that, in reasonable estimations, would serve to aid rather than replace medical professionals. Demonstrably, one broad AI diagnostic system sits in recent memory of some oncologists as a stunning failure that highlights the limitations of AI-enabled healthcare at present. From its early inception, IBM's AI-driven Watson supercomputer was hailed by the company as harnessing the power to revolutionize cancer care. Beginning in 2013, IBM initiated partnerships with leading medical institutions renowned for their research in oncology such as the MD Anderson Cancer Center at the University of Texas, the Memorial Sloan-Kettering Cancer Center in New York, and the University of North Carolina's Lineberger Comprehensive Cancer Center. IBM bought a multitude of competitor companies and spent millions in order to train Watson on crucial medical data including biomedical literature, patient histories and data, billing records, and medical histories. Although Watson had some success at the University North Carolina in identifying relevant clinical trials for patients and suggesting potential treatments based on its ability to ingest peer-reviewed biomedical literature, Watson was deemed a stunning failure and scrapped by MD Anderson in early 2016 following missed deadlines, a series of fruitless pilot projects, and continuous changes to the types of cancer that would harness Watson's focus. Watson's problems at MD Anderson involved a limited ability to understand and suggest actionable insights from the medical data it ingested was made worse by fragmentary clinical data and a lack of evidentiary support in the studies it analyzed. Costing MD Anderson over 62 million dollars before its collapse, investing in Watson proved a remarkable blunder for the cancer research center [12]. A former manager at IBM asserts a further reason as to why the project failed miserably in its lofty efforts to transform oncology. In his estimation, IBM "turned the marketing engine loose without controlling how to build and construct a product" [5]. Topol summarizes that while "there is certainly potential for computing to make a major difference [in medicine and oncology more broadly]... so far there has been minimal delivery on the promise." Topol contends that the difficulty in assembly and aggregation of data has been underestimated, not just by Watson, but a myriad of tech companies venturing into healthcare [5]. The hype surrounding AI-enabled healthcare tools and indeed, the fortunes at stake, leads technology producers, marketers, commentators, investors, patients, and medical specialists to overestimate the speed of development and delivery of AI systems and, can result in ungrounded and uncritical conceptions of their potential to make significant, comprehensive impacts on medical care and of the liabilities these technologies can incur.

4.3 Defining standards and ensuring quality access to care in a context marked by enduring health inequities

Beyond a modest view for the rates of widespread AI development and deployment, potential of instantiations of AI-enabled healthcare also brings other critical considerations and challenges to the fore. One of the current challenges hampering AI-enabled approaches for routine use in clinical settings involves the lack of appropriate coherency regarding what constitutes standardization regarding these tools. The disparate development of tools utilizing machine learning techniques has produced a paradigm in which the same clinical question is addressed by separate systems developed in independent institutions. Validated on particular and distinct datasets or samples, these systems may produce different outputs, which can ultimately result in differing clinical recommendations and patient outcomes [10]. For example, pathologists can disagree whether a biopsy sample taken from a breast tissue is cancerous, which some studies suggest has contributed to an over-diagnosis of breast cancer. The subtle abnormalities exhibited by small, early-stage cancers are particularly difficult to diagnose. This issue extends beyond breast cancer to diagnosing melanomas, thyroid cancer, and prostate cancer. Existing clinical disagreement over what constitutes cancer may lead to cancer screening AI tools that mimic a tendency for over-diagnosis [13].

When applying an AI-driven tool in a clinical scenario, clinicians and other health professionals across institutions and national borders must have definitive assurances of scalable clinical standardization to deliver appropriate quality of care. Consequently, this requires international collaboration that must necessarily involve technology producers, clinical specialists, and regulatory bodies. Moreover, ensuring all patients have access to state of the art, AI-driven healthcare remains a significant challenge. Similar to other new technologies, experts predict that AI-enabled medical tools will be extremely costly for health institutions initially and will gradually decrease in expense over time. Given the potential of, for example, more timely diagnosis and improved disease monitoring made possible by AI tools, patients being treated at medical centers able to afford AI resources are likely to experience better health outcomes than those at institutions without the financial means to invest in these expensive resources. In addition to possessing considerable economic resources, medical centers may also need to train health professionals in the workings and use of these tools, which presents another potential hurdle to the widespread deployment of these systems.

Furthermore, the U.S.-based research of both professor of medicine and clinical surgery at the University of Illinois, Robert A. Winn, and anthropologist Kadija

Ferryman of the Data and Society Research Institute, enjoins them to contextualize AI-driven success stories in medicine—especially in the realm of cancer care—against the backdrop of enduring health disparities in the United States. Although health expenditures in the U.S. are colossal with healthcare constituting more than 18% of the United States' gross domestic product (climbing more than 10 percentage points since 1975), increased healthcare spending has not corresponded to improved healthcare outcomes across population groups in the U.S. [5]. Ferryman and Winn stress the sobering fact that people of color continue to have disproportionately higher incidence and mortality rates for multiple cancers (among them: kidney, breast, cervical, and prostate cancer) as they pose the following question: "As big data comes to cancer care, how can we ensure that it is addressing issues of equity, and that these new technologies will not further entrench disparities in cancer?" [14]. Winn and Ferryman join other medical researchers in arguing that not only does a shift in increased usage of medical AI tools necessitate population-representative data accessibility coupled with regulatory paradigms to ensure standardization and quality, but it also requires prioritizing healthcare equity, ethical health mandates, and inclusivity [15].

For example, Winn and Ferryman bring attention to how such a shift would impact the clinical responsibilities of health professionals. They reason that due to the nature of clinical care, clinicians must be able to assess, understand, and explain machine learning-driven systems to patients. Consequently this necessitates a certain level of transparency in how these systems are trained, developed, and produce outputs; these systems cannot be fully "black-boxed." With the capacity of these technologies to refigure clinicians' responsibilities, Winn and Ferryman echo a chorus of legal scholars who forewarn that a more robust integration of AI tools in clinical settings may incur both a transformation of the patient-doctor relationship as well as a reconceptualization of the regulations surrounding malpractice. Winn and Ferryman further contend that a shift in clinicians' liabilities and obligations to demystify AI systems for patients may incur higher stakes for patients with "limited access to high quality clinical care, limited health literacy, earned mistrust of medical providers, and those individuals who may be exposed to interpersonal and institutional racism and discrimination in their healthcare encounters" [14]. They argue that it is critical that the potential ramifications for vulnerable patients due to the integration of AI technology in the clinic be not only acknowledged but also, consistently and intentionally managed. Together, these aforementioned challenges consist of only a small sampling of the issues that must be addressed before a successful, widespread adoption of AI-driven medical tools can be undertaken.

5. Methods and methodology

This chapter is informed by and enlists textual, ethnographic, and other qualitative data that the author has collected in undertaking a broad examination of the legal, political, and ethical imperatives surrounding the development of AI-driven systems for healthcare and for oncology, specifically. This study attends to patient reception of the development and deployment of these systems as well as patients' perceptions and willingness to participate in health-related AI development by sharing medical data necessary to train and improve these systems with public and private entities engaged in developing them.

This analysis draws upon qualitative research methods including textual and content analysis of academic literature reviews, general audience media, and industry-oriented publications. This study was further augmented by an in-depth, semi-structured interview protocol. In addition to attending cancer patient conferences, talks, and support groups, the author conducted interviews with 40 relevant stakeholders. The approximately 15 hours of observation and 40 interviews were undertaken for the first 11 months of 2019. Interlocutors included cancer patients and their caregivers, cancer patient advocates, directors and specialists at cancer care nonprofits, technologists employed at firms developing AI tools for oncology, and clinicians. The interview corpus of this study includes 9 U.S. citizens, 29 U.K. citizens, and 5 citizens from the European Union. Interviews were primarily conducted in cities located in Northern California in the U.S. as well as in London and Cambridgeshire in the U.K.

Among the interview corpus, 28 individuals are cancer patients who were actively undergoing treatment or who were in remission at the time of the interview. Seven patients were in remission at the time the interviews were conducted and the remaining 21 patients are currently receiving treatment for their cancers. Twenty-four of the patients were born between 1939 and 1960.The four remaining patients were born after 1983, the youngest patient interviewed was born in 1990. The majority of the patients interviewed are retired from the workforce having had previous careers as secretaries, telecom and systems engineers, insurance salesmen, military logisticians, child-care providers, librarians, photographers, teachers, and small-business owners. At the time of the interviews, patients in the interview corpus who were in the workforce had employment as data scientists, teachers, lab technicians, and engineers. Those with employment were generally employed as part-time employees as a result of their continuing treatments. Other patients were stay-at-home parents and one patient is a doctoral student. When asked about socioeconomic status, most patients considered themselves to be middle-class. The patients in this interview corpus are of white, European descent although the interview corpus as a whole and the ethnographic work that supplements this study involved patients, advocates, and healthcare professionals from other ethnic and racial backgrounds. The patients interviewed possessed a multitude of different cancer diagnoses. Three of the patients interviewed had received a diagnosis of colorectal cancer; six had received a diagnosis of breast cancer; two had received a diagnosis of cervical cancer; six had received a diagnosis of bladder cancer; five had received a diagnosis of prostate cancer; seven had received lymphoma diagnoses; four had received a diagnosis of myeloma; and, one patient had received a diagnosis of skin cancer (several patients had developed multiple cancers).

Three individuals within this interview corpus are clinicians. Two of these clinicians are senior oncologists with extensive experience working at illustrious cancer research hospitals in the United Kingdom, Ireland, Italy, and the United States. The final clinician is completing their initial rotation-years as a pediatrician at a premiere research hospital on the west coast of the United States; this clinician previously earned a doctorate degree in medical anthropology. Their dissertation research studied patient data-sharing and patient reception of self-tracking approaches to medical care. Seven interviews were conducted with data scientists, bioinformaticians, and start-up founders who work or previously worked at a U.K. and U.S.-based AI oncology-related start-up.

The remaining five interlocutors comprising this interview corpus are trained cancer patient advocates. One of these patient advocates is a U.K. citizen and the remaining four are U.S. citizens. All are based in California although three of them occasionally serve as advocates and patient ethicists for projects at renowned cancer research institutes in other U.S. states. One of these advocates is a licensed nurse practitioner with experience in global health consultancy; this advocate currently serves as the program director of a nonprofit cancer care center and clinic located in a Northern Californian metropolis. Another cancer patient advocate in this corpus has nearly three decades of experience and has earned several awards and accolades for her advocacy work. Previously, this advocate was employed as a patient advocate and advisor at an eminent national cancer support organization and is presently employed as a senior patient navigator with a focus on multicultural patient support at a California nonprofit that primarily caters to local, low-income women of color who have received cancer diagnoses although the organization remains open patients of all backgrounds. In her role, this advocate guides patients through treatment, clinical trial options and hospital visits; assists patients with insurance forms and other medical paperwork; and provides patients with counseling and much needed psycho-social support. This advocate regularly serves on cancer patient advocate conference committees, counsels researchers seeking to work with cancer patients, and acts as a grant reviewer for emerging research ventures. The three remaining advocates have diverse employment histories in the fields of marketing, graphic design, emergency medicine, and nonprofit leadership. For nearly 15 years, these trained cancer survivor advocates with expertise in research and patient communication have worked with national and local advocacy organizations serving on survivorship and research committees for various academic, nonprofit, and governmental organizations. They frequently serve as research partners and advocates on scientific review committees and act as grant reviewers for emerging university-led research projects in the state of California. They also serve on clinical trials advisory committees as advocate observers, patient advisors, and stakeholder reviewers in partnership with state and national research bodies as well as national cancer research organizations including the National Institutes of Health, the American Cancer Society, the Department of Defense, and the Susan G. Komen Foundation. These advocates routinely volunteer at local nonprofits as helpline attendees and peer mentors to cancer patients currently undergoing treatment.

Coagulating and analyzing this qualitative data, this chapter offers insight into the perceptions and concerns some cancer patients (i.e., particularly those identifying as middle class and of European descent), patient advocates, and clinicians abiding in the Home Counties of the U.K. and Northern Californian metropolises possess regarding both the deployment of AI systems for oncology as well as sharing health data with public and private entities for the purpose of developing these systems. Complementing the textual and ethnographic data, the interview work conducted enumerates popular dispositions toward biomedical technological development for oncology within the socially stratified societies of the U.S. and the U.K. as well as refracts the particular exigencies of pursuing cancer treatments within the two nations' contrasting healthcare systems.

Researchers studying the social and technical valences of AI continue to insist upon the foundational legitimacy and, indeed, the value of studying popular conceptions of machine learning-driven systems. Public perceptions contribute to the fashioning of the material and discursive realities these systems act upon and within and furthermore constitute collective contestations of the political realities, ethical liabilities, and financial viabilities immanent to the social production of these technological systems. Correspondingly, Monteescu and Elish contend that "When it comes to understanding the impact of AI, the social perceptions of a technology's capabilities are equally important to technical definitions. Elsewhere we have observed that non-expert understandings of AI are often shaped by marketing rhetoric, which sometimes suggests capabilities that are not yet technically possible. For many developers of AI systems, this potential fuzziness is 'not a bug but a feature,' so to speak. The public perception of AI is often leveraged to drum up excitement or stand in for a range of automated technologies that haven't yet become fully actualized. The fluctuating understandings of AI will not be universally resolved, and so it is necessary to account for the consequences of AI as defined through both technical definitions and social representations" [16]. Public trust, knowledge, and perception of health data-sharing and AI development and deployment will undoubtedly influence how governments, health organizations, and corporate entities continue to debate, contest, insist on, and invest in AI viability for medical usage. For this reason, public perceptions may also impact the material development of these systems (e.g., via a collective willingness or unwillingness to use these systems for medical treatment or engage in health data-sharing for AI development); the regulatory mandates and other frameworks of standardization, equity, and accountability pursued in their wake; the funding and long-term economic feasibility of these systems; and perhaps even the meaning of what medical care can or should constitute.

6. Understanding patient perceptions of AI-driven systems for healthcare

This chapter presents an analytic overview of: the extent of knowledge a sample of U.S. and U.K. patients possess regarding AI systems for oncology and oncology-related drug development as well as healthcare, more broadly. Similar to other recent studies, the qualitative research that this discussion derives from indicates that general public audiences (inclusive of cancer patients) continue to possess varied notions of not only what constitutes AI, but also what capabilities these AI systems hold and the extent of proficiency with which they presently perform them. With varied (although certainly increasing) levels of sophistication, cancer patients (as evidenced in the interview sample) are questioning what potential ramifications patients should be aware of, and potentially concerned about, regarding the usage of AI systems for healthcare and oncology. They question what emotive and affective positions they should take with regard to AI Certainly, patients possess divergent understandings of both when and how this technology may impact or augment the standard of care within oncology that directs recommended treatment paths and contributes to patient outcomes. Nevertheless, many are attentive to the limitations of their current knowledge regarding these systems. In consequence, patients are questioning how they can stay informed, what constitutes trustworthy sources from which they can glean accurate and legible information, and what specific types of inquiries should they be attending to.

In order for healthcare technologies to be effectively responsive to patients' needs, it is evident that institutions, persons, and entities involved in developing instruments that can affect cancer patients' quality of care not only assess patients' present knowledge and perceptions of emerging technology, but also heed and address their resultant questions and concerns. With a preponderant focus on analyzing the interview data the author has collected, this chapter assesses the express knowledge, perceptions, and suggestions a sample of U.S. and U.K. patients possess regarding AI systems for oncology and oncology drug development. Specifically, this chapter enumerates three primary analytical axes in attending to this dataset: cancer patients' perception of AI systems for oncology; their willingness to contribute to the development of the efficacy of these systems and AI-drug development via medical data-sharing; the concerns they bear regarding both the deployment and integration of these systems as well as health data-sharing for the aforementioned purposes; and finally, the recommendations patients and relevant experts are proposing for building accountability measures to ensure both safe usage and improve patient trust.

6.1 Patients' expressed levels of knowledge

In characterizing the knowledge the patient interlocutors comprising the interview corpus possessed at the time the interviews were conducted, it is principally important to register that the vast majority of these cancer patients had no formal or professional training in regards to these systems. While four of the patients offered examples demonstrating how they currently utilize or previously utilized machine learning systems in their employment, the remaining number (86% of the patient interlocutors) had no professional experience with these systems and learned about AI primarily through general audience media. All things considered, the interview data are largely representative then of not just modes of public perception but lay opinion. All of the patients, with the exception of one, registered having heard the term of AI and exhibited a capacity to grasp the foundations of its most basic principles. These interlocutors, moreover, often went on to demonstrate the applicability of AI tools or machine learning-driven systems within healthcare contexts. Furthermore, when offering examples, patient interlocutors chiefly cited examples from both oncology and general practitioner diagnostics. Those who demonstrated a familiarity of the application of machine learning systems to oncology most frequently cited its current applicability to pathology, medical robotics, and multi-omics data-handling. Five patient interlocutors within the interview corpus related having previously prepared reports or presentations in which they offered an introductory overview of AI and AI applicability to oncology for either cancer patients and advocates, or otherwise general public audiences.

Unsurprisingly, the interviews exhibited a wide range of patient articulations of the foundational aspects of AI systems. For example, when asked what they knew about AI, one patient insisted that they knew "very little"; "I would assume it has something to do with algorithms. In [our support] group, we've talked about how there might be some algorithms that can be used for diagnostic tools for GP's. To me, I don't know if this is right, but AI has to do with data-handling. There's so much data out in this world and we have to think about how are we going to make it useful." After explaining that they first learned about the principles of AI from early science fiction novels (such as Isaac Asimov's *I, Robot*), one patient defined AI in the following terms: "Well, I would say it is, basically, a computer that is capable of interpreting input, and making deductions from input that it is given. Obviously, the way it responds to that is being presumably programmed by a human being. But, I believe that computers, or at least AI, are capable of taking it beyond that, they're capable of learning from the basic information they're been given and building on that." Another patient interlocutor explained: "Well, to my mind, AI is programming a computer of some sort to take various in-puts and to learn from them, basically. So if you got say, a visual system—cancers on an x-ray for example, you would have a system that you could teach. Say, put through a number positives or a number negatives of say a thousand scans and maybe a hundred of those are positive and you teach it to compare it to the negative ones and identify which ones are positive. Then you can leave it on its own to work by itself from that point on. Y'know once you are satisfied that it's strike-rate is sufficient. You can leave it to its own devices. That's how I kind of look at medical AI anyway. I also think AI is very much a black box, just from what I've seen on the telly. You set it going but you don't necessarily understand how it's doing it. *[laughing]*... Whether that's true or not, I don't know. But that's my perception of it from the popular media I guess...I have no idea just how much AI is actually out there and performing at the moment, if you see what I mean. How far it's come; how much use there is for it at present; whether it still remains a largely experimental field." These three explanations offer a triangulation of the amount of knowledge and levels of coherency the majority of the cancer patients interviewed expressed to the author. Many could give a relatively clear articulation of how the elementary facets of machine learning or of how AI algorithms function. Typically, this sample of patients demonstrated that these systems function to process vast amounts of data, that with appropriate engineering and sufficient data training sets these algorithms can be "trained" to identify relevant variables as outputs, and that AI can be applied to medical data and have potential use for oncology.

Excluding the four patient interlocutors who have professional training in and experience with AI systems, patients related that they had arrived at their current level of knowledge through general audience media. In particular, all of the remaining patient interlocutors cited two primary sources from which they derived knowledge regarding these systems. All related that they had learned about AI from journalistic sources and accounts they encountered via print media such as a local, national, international, or specialized newspapers (e.g., a business newspaper or magazine) and digital news platforms. Secondly, all related that they had gained an initial introduction to or a partial familiarity with the general principles of AI via speculative accounts found in genre fiction sources such as science fiction texts, films, and television series. Some indicated that accounts concerning AI in speculative fiction or journalistic sources sparked a personal interest in these systems and their development; these patient interlocutors explained that they further bolstered their knowledge through nonfiction texts about AI development and applicability. Otherwise, patients related that they had further learned about AI via friends, spouses, or relatives who have professional involvement with AI Some reported having been informed by existing government reports (e.g., the U.K.'s 2018 House of Lords Report on Artificial Intelligence) that they were initially made aware of from journalistic sources. A small number of patient interlocutors indicated that they also learned about AI via their involvement in patient support groups or patient advocacy work (including oncology-related conferences and involvement with medical research auditing).

6.2 Patients' general perceptions of AI

Overwhelming, the cancer patients interviewed for this study held positive perceptions and opinions for the development of AI systems for oncology. With the exception of one patient interlocutor who admitted no knowledge and no opinions of these tools, the patient interlocutors comprising the interview corpus voiced hope for the relevancy and potential for AI development and application for medicine. Continuously, these patients insisted that as a "useful tool," "able to catch things humans can't," AI systems would be a "step forward" inasmuch as they "will make things better" by "improv[ing] speed and quality of data analysis." As one patient put it: "we've been waiting for a faster identification of things and this can only help." Others noted with pronounced optimism that these tools may "reduce workloads" for medical professionals such as doctors and nurses. One patient mused that perhaps such systems could combat clinical biases and bigotry through objective and accurate data-handling; a view that has been critiqued by social researchers of technology as misguided. "Generally," another patient concluded, "I think tech advances are a good thing." Another interlocutor echoed this statement, adding: "It sounds great and I think it will give people confidence and perhaps a better chance at survival."

Patients who possessed professional training or work experience in developing and deploying AI systems expressed similar hope and positivity about AI-enabled healthcare. One patient who works with AI tools as a lab technician within the context of drug development remarked that AI tools are "something in development that can be really useful, especially for handling patient data and especially genomics data… It's really good for things that have a clear 'yes' or 'no' and beyond that there are always new improvements, new features to improve the algorithms with… If [AI tools for oncology] allow for the use of certain data like mutations and other genomics data, they could provide more confidence in the use of AI for cancer treatment predictions." Two other patients, with tangential familiarity with AI systems given their respective professions as a statistician and systems engineer asserted that AI presented "a lot to be gained" and especially holds promise for the improvement of diagnostics. The systems engineer asserted his belief that, used in the arena of oncology, AI tools may "bring reliable indications for decisions that don't get made or get lost in communication."

Notably, many of the patient interlocutors interviewed characterized their perceptions of AI tools as thoroughly secondary and overshadowed by the currency and pervasiveness of popular teleological narratives of technology that cast technological development as both heroic and as "inevitable progress." Concerning AI-enabled healthcare, patients frequently conceded: "It's the way of the future." In turn, some expressed that their conceptions of the inevitability of technological progression (in this instance, made manifest by AI tools for healthcare) encouraged feelings that "[The prospect of AI-enabled oncology] is exciting, but a little scary." In other words, among declarations of the hope regarding the potential of AI, many patients voiced tepid fears in relation to offering their assessments of AI tools given their (and potentially others') beliefs in the potential marginality of their own social locations—as, for instance, elders and, more broadly, as cancer patients. What would often begin as self-aware statements relating limited abilities to stay current with the seeming swiftness of many technological shifts and innovations, would in many interviews lead to remarks through which patients would minimize their relevancy and position to offer opinions, thoughts, or concerns about AI "Are we doomed?" one patient asked, "I don't know. All I know is that [AI development] is unstoppable and frankly…you can't put yesterday's values on tomorrow." Another insisted: "Everything is moving forward and does move forward. Why should this be any different? It's how we live, and maybe we just need to get on and accept it." Others voiced that regardless of the advancements in AI, they feel they are "too old" to "keep up" and described feeling as if they are suspended in a paradigm of being left behind with regard to their technological knowledge and savviness and have accepted this predicament as "their lot": "Things move quickly and I've switched off." In addition to age, patients pointed to their diagnosis and the rigorousness of their therapies as preventing them from seeing the future of AI development for oncology as pertinent to them. Patients interviewed in the middle of treatment cycles voiced a similar sentiment of being too sick to "keep up" or of not feeling capable of appropriately assessing how it would affect the future of oncology, let alone themselves and others. In fact, some patients asserted confidently: "[These tools] won't affect me."

Patients who were familiar with AI due to the nature of their professional employment admitted that while they firmly supported the technology's use and development with great hope, in their view, these systems generally remain "under-developed and under-utilized." "Changes are happening," these patients declared, "but slowly." Likewise, one patient advocate related: "I've been hearing a lot about [AI tools for oncology] at conferences and it sounds wonderful but I haven't seen it materialize yet in hospitals and clinics."

In summary, some patients (often those with lay knowledge of AI systems) consider AI systems for oncology and medicine to be developing at a rapid rate and intertwine this conception of rapid technological development with a notion of "natural" and "inevitable" technological progression against which they would unfavorably compare their age and health status as inversely related. In this view, their age and health status become barriers that immobilize their capacity to stay informed and interested in technological development. This logic perhaps serves as a basis for elaborating insecurities about whether they have an appropriate ability to speak lucidly or incisively about AI tools for oncology which, at times, results in a firm belief that they should not concern themselves with forming critical views and voicing judgments about the subject.

Beyond highlighting contrasting conceptions of the pace of AI development, patients framed their enthusiasm regarding AI systems for oncology with statements conceding a general awareness that technological transition may produce vulnerabilities and risks for patients and medical staff. Despite widely expressed optimism, a majority of patients voiced that shifting to a greater use of AI tools for oncology and medicine may subject patients to additional risk for medical errors or mishaps. "There's always room for errors and mistakes," as one patient mused. "Errors," another patient conceded, "are inevitable and it takes time to perfect technology. That's progression. We learn by mistakes, sadly." Further epitomizing this appraisal, a patient familiar with machine learning techniques explained: "If used for the benefit of mankind [sic], I am absolutely onboard for this tech. Bring it on. But forcing learning when the data isn't there, isn't the right thing to do." In other words, despite an embrace of narratives of technological progression, patients voiced a desire for cautious progression of AI tools and emphasized the potential human costs of technological innovation and initial deployment.

Moreover, many patients indicated that they believe such tools may, in the future, produce some level of job insecurity for certain doctors and medical staff (e.g., radiologists, pathologists). Still, those who voiced this issue noted that they prioritized manifesting better health outcomes for patients over maintaining employment for medical professionals able to produce less satisfactory health outcomes. Others related that they believe that these tools will not encroach on the necessity of the roles of medical professionals or threaten their employment prospects but will instead produce "a major sea-change for the medical industry," the consequence of which being that doctors and other medical staff will "need to be retrained or receive additional training."

Finally, a small minority of patients experience the prospect of AI-enabled healthcare as shrouded in confusion and potential conspiracy. "I have concerns about it," one patient admitted, "but only in a SciFi-horror film kind of way which is based on ignorance and a certain amount of misinformation." Other patients related more earnest concerns about AI tools for healthcare regarding potential issues of developers' nefarious intent, consolidated power, and misguided objectives. One patient confessed these fears in the following manner: "In my way of understanding, ultimately, AI will be writing the software itself. And that's where it goes out of control because from what I've seen, personally, and to the present day, software engineers have a lot of power, a lot of power! And the people who write the software...they could conceal things, you get an unscrupulous one. Ninety-nine percent, I'm sure, are perfectly legitimate, but it only needs one or two unscrupulous ones who can put bugs in software. And it worries me that, as I say, ultimately, that software won't be written by humans—the software itself will be interpreted and written by AI and I'm sure that's ultimately where we're going." Other patients voiced wariness that there exists far too much control over the development and deployment of AI systems "in the hands of too few." They stressed the need to democratize relations of power relating to how private entities and corporate structures consolidate the decision-making power over how and which issues are tackled with AI tools and consequently, how these tools are designed and implemented across sectors within and outside of medicine (e.g., the workings of financial services companies and investment banks or the political encroachment and monopolistic tendencies of tech mammoths such as Amazon, Google, and Facebook). Some patients' portends remained vaguely sketched: "Like all tech, evil men get behind it and we see the bad side of everything...Insert *Blade Runner* quote here."

In parallel, other patients declared that although they felt generally optimistic about the prospects of AI developments for healthcare, they underscored a desire for these technologies "to improve quality of life, not extend it." One patient admitted, "I don't want AI to cure cancer in order for people to live forever." Evidently, one patient advocate insisted, "The promise of Big Data is confusing for patients." Patient interlocutors with technical expertise and familiarity with AI systems expressed their bafflement over other patients' and public figures' confusions regarding these systems. One of these patients voiced his frustrations regarding the philosophical or imaginative fears some lay members of the public have: "I don't understand why people think it's some *Doctor Who*-Take-Over-the World syndrome!...most people in the last 30-40 years, would have used computing techniques of some sort to break down their spreadsheet or whatever. Conceptually, I don't see a great difference between AI and that....I can't wrap my head around why people think it's some sort of SciFi, *Doctor Who* thing or, why they think it's something that's been invented last week by Amazon. It's been around thirty years or so and the math has been around for one hundred years! And secondly, they've been doing it all their lives!" While this patient thought it might aid others without expertise to understand what he understood as the banalities of AI by drawing conceptual comparisons to more simple computing properties, another suggested confusions and conspiracy theories could be attributed to idiomatic decisions. He explained: "I feel, sort of working in that area, that we should stop talking about artificial intelligence and talk more about machine learning or statistical learning. Talk about something different from artificial intelligence because when people think about that they think of Arnold Schwarzenegger and *The Terminator.* In fact, statistical techniques, which are not strictly artificial intelligence, have been around for 30 years. There's all sorts of techniques that we rely on that have been around for decades." Together, their comments demonstrate the diverse range of general apperceptions of what these technologies might accomplish, how who develops and deploys these technologies may impact healthcare systems (including patients and medical professionals), and how popular depictions of and professional experience with AI tools contribute to contrasting notions and appraisals of their influence, application, and current state of development.

7. Patient concerns regarding the development, integration, and deployment of AI tools in healthcare contexts

Despite varying levels of expertise and general knowledge, the patient interlocutors interviewed for this study expressed overlapping concerns regarding the development, integration, and deployment of AI tools for oncology and for use within healthcare contexts more broadly. Patients regularly articulated three core areas of concern regarding issues of regulatory oversight, development and training matters, as well as issues of standardization and integration. Together, these common concerns demonstrate how patients are ingesting existing reports of unintended effects and social risks AI systems across different sectors have resulted in. Moreover, they exhibit how patients are envisioning and responding to the potential for AI technologies to produce instances of medical error and harm.

7.1 Patient concerns regarding the need for regulatory oversight

The fulcrum of patient interlocutors' anxieties concern the need for regulatory oversight of AI tools. This issue materialized as a constant chorus for patients across nearly every interview. One mode in which this issue was raised was as a desire for a "human buffer" or a technical, medical expert between these systems and patients. Patients stressed that, beyond issues of efficacy, they were concerned that health providers might attempt to thoroughly replace "the human element of care" from medical contexts. "Regarding automation and AI techniques" one patient explained, "I think it is comforting to have a human around you. Or, to have a human be the bridge between robotics and the person, the impersonal screen and the person... I think personally it's still nice to get some human element of care." To ensure the retainment of this experience of care, patients enumerated preferences for trained medical experts to explain how these systems work, to remain available and present, and to oversee the results that these systems produce in real-time. Furthermore, patients fear the possibility of these systems to possess the power of executive decision-making. They instead stressed the need to limit the function of these systems to auxiliary tools that enable medical professionals and patients to make better-informed medical decisions. One patient elaborated: "As for [AI systems] making decisions, I don't think it's the way to go. I think it should be the way it's done now, they give you all the options and the patient can make the decisions. Not the machine or anyone else."

Even more frequently, patient interlocutors articulated the need for regulatory agencies and bodies to effectuate heightened oversight, greater legal accountability, and guaranteed quality control of these systems as a mandatory precondition to ensuring the prevention of medical error. In order to establish the responsible use of these systems within medical contexts, patients asserted that these systems cannot be introduced into clinical settings without appropriate regulatory safeguards. A patient interlocutor articulated this issue as such: "I don't think it can just be done and introduced and used. I think safeguards have got to be put in place and monitored. But who does that? I don't know." Other patients voiced misgivings concerning the current lack of regulations because of the existing confusion of when robust regulatory schemes will be introduced and how they will operate. Particularly, patients are concerned with how regulatory schemes will be organized to arrange the necessary flexibility, international collaboration, and enforcement capacity to assure both the optimization of these systems and patient safety.

7.2 Patient concerns regarding the facets of AI development

In addition to concerns about the establishment of robust regulatory networks, patient interlocutors were also perturbed by unresolved several facets of current AI development. Foremost, given AI systems' reliance on training datasets to improve the accuracy and efficiency of its outputs, patients stressed developers of AI medical tools are faced with crucial mandates regarding the assemblage of training datasets. Patient interlocutors stressed that ensuring regulatory usage and patient trust is fundamentally contingent upon developers' abilities to guarantee the accuracy, completeness, and representativeness of their datasets. As one patient warned, "forcing learning when the data isn't there, isn't the right thing to do." In questioning the potential for this technology to address health disparities or further entrench them, some patients raised concerns of how researchers and developers are grappling with the limitations of existing health data. Often these data are representative of only a small portion of world's population. Patients fear that if AI systems are trained on inadequate or unrepresentative data, these systems could potentially reify medical insights (as well as produce medicines and outcomes) with limited efficacy. Emphasizing the need to compile population-representative datasets, one patient disclosed: "My other concern with machine learning or AI, it's sort of like that old saying for computers: 'Garbage in, Garbage out': to make sure you are getting the best training sets from African Americans and Asian Americans and Native Americans and not just Americans but all races [across different populations]... because that's sort of the big picture. That is the problem with clinical trials in the U.S.—you get a bunch of white people! So racial diversity [is needed] and are you getting enough participants across all age groups?" To assemble representative, comprehensive, and accurate datasets, patients further asserted that health researchers and AI medical tool developers should be engaging in more collaborative research rather than "working in silos" and aim to include multiple kinds of health data including multi-omics data and even non-biological or environmental data or multiple data points derived from multiple sources and perimeters. By the same token, patients were adamant that AI systems for medical use must be able to be updated to integrate new forms of health data. For example, one patient mused, that if an AI system functioned to predict health outcomes for patients with a certain cancer on a specific treatment protocol, it may run into issues if new therapies are discovered and become standard. Given this scenario, he explained, "the relevance of the model becomes less significant. So there are issues around that. The earlier you are in the interference of data—that is, the ability to learn outcomes against base data is hugely, hugely relevant." Correspondingly, patients were concerned about the abilities of AI models to be able to be responsive to additional information, changes and updates within health contexts. How will that be ensured, they asked? And how will the regulatory process account for this given that these systems should be retrained often?

Patients also questioned the efficacy of AI development given the relative homogeneity of developers. Some patient interlocutors questioned whether emerging AI-driven health technologies might only be fully responsive to and efficacious for the demographic groups resembling developers. These patients worry that as the tech industry is dominated by affluent to middle-class, cis-, white, male developers, the questions, issues, and systems developers are currently pursuing might bear the (un) conscious markings of developers' particular systemic privileges, interests, politics, desires, and bodies [17]. These patients reason that the needs, worldviews, and commitments of those developing technological instruments will inevitably influence how these instruments will take shape in the world. Compounded by the troubling homogeneity of the tech industry, these patients foresee that these technologies have the potential to embody prejudices, unconscious blindspots, or inherent bias that could result in "unintended harm" that disproportionately affects the most vulnerable in society. Patients stressed the need for "diverse developing teams" who will hold "diversity of viewpoints" and attend to their technologies' capabilities to reinforce structural inequities and unjust psychological biases to produce harm for patients. Their comments are heedful of the extent to which developers are concerned with constructing tools that function to oppose apathy, greed, and inequity. As one patient contended: "Your tech needs to include and account for everyone or you will create more barriers to quality care. It's about making sure you don't leave certain patients in the 'Dark Age' and giving all patients the right treatments for the strongest chance at survival."

7.3 Patient concerns regarding health system integration and access

Furthermore, patients remain troubled by concerns regarding standardization, health system integration, and unequal access to leading-edge medical care. Some patient interlocutors voiced doubts regarding the ability of their current health system to integrate and implement the use of these tools in a successful, rapid, and straightforward manner. As a result of predicaments stemming from its bureaucratic structure and mishaps related to its ability to securely manage health data, some U.K. patients held misgivings about the feasibility of the National Health Service to manage a transition to widespread, systematic use of cutting-edge, AI-driven medical tools. Comparatively, U.S. patients frequently voiced integration concerns relating to how the largely for-profit and privatized U.S. healthcare system results in unequal access to standard of care and even basic health services. As the healthcare landscape in the U.S. remains stunningly rife with inequities, patients fear a potential worsening of the existing unequal implementation and access to AI-driven systems for medical use. Accordingly, U.S. patients asked: what hospitals and medical centers have the resources to launch and integrate this technology for patients' benefits? What patients will be denied access because of factors such as geographic location, healthcare provider, hospital availability, and insurance issues? How will this further entrench existing healthcare inequities? "While some patients might have access [to cutting-edge AI tools for oncology] through tertiary centers and university research hospitals, what's happening at local clinics and hospitals?" one U.S. patient asked. "How will standardization play out?" she continued, "We have to make sure that people—that everybody—has access to it and that's not the case here." Another U.S. cancer patient advocate further elaborated: "Everyone is thinking it is promising and that it will come our way. My concern is that it is broadly accepted to be covered by public systems. We see a lot of disparities in terms of what public insurance like Medicare and Medicaid will cover versus what private insurance will cover. So my fear is that we are going to have two tiers." Patient interlocutors comprising this interview corpus recognize that issues surrounding financial resources and incentives as well as individual health system's bureaucratic and political structures will contribute to the ease or difficulty of systematic integration of AI tools for medicine. In turn, they reason that this may affect unequal access to the most efficacious care and thus, contribute to the further entrenchment of existing healthcare inequities.

8. Understanding patient perceptions regarding data-sharing for AI and drug development research

Access to health datasets is a crucial factor in enabling oncology-specific drug development and AI systems research. This section examines patient responses and concerns regarding sharing their health data for these aforementioned purposes. Together, the comments of this sample of cancer patient interlocutors compose an opening through which to understand some patients' perceptions, misconceptions, and misgivings regarding sharing their health data. Moreover, their responses exhibit variance in both existing knowledge of cancer patients and the extent to which they express a desire to be involved in the advancement of proposed AI systems for oncology and oncology drug development vis-a-vis data-sharing.

8.1 Data-sharing and research participation: concerns and caveats

Virtually all of the cancer patients interviewed for this study expressed both general enthusiasm and an overall willingness to be involved in oncology drug development and oncology AI tool advancement in some capacity. Furthermore, nearly 22% of the patients comprising the interview corpus indicated that they trust the regulatory schemes and ethical parameters that currently guide public and private entities involved in research enough to be willing to share their medical data for research purposes without any additional conditions or specific requests beyond these existing mandates. The potential for various issues pertaining to data security, storage, targeted surveillance, as well as risks of data re-identification and discrimination, did not inhibit these patients' desire to contribute to oncology drug and AI development research. In their view, these potential complications did not present an undue risk to them given the existing frameworks of ethical and legal protections regarding research.

Nevertheless, the remaining portion of patient interlocutors held concerns and caveats potent enough to potentially prevent them from agreeing to participate in research. These patients presented a series of considerations that they specifically want corporate researchers to address in order for them to feel comfortable enough to agree to contribute health data for a private entities' (e.g., pharmaceutical or biotech companies) efforts to conduct research regardless of their affiliations with medical research institutes or university research centers. Notably, however, when presented with a hypothetical scenario in which a university or medical research institute was conducting research without corporate collaboration (exclusive of funding) nearly all patients were willing to offer their medical data without any major caveats although a small number insisted that their willingness to share their data would be affected by corporate sponsorship in this scenario.

8.2 Concerns regarding data security and patient privacy

Most commonly, patient interlocutors declared that their primary concern with respect to sharing medical data for research purposes pertains to issues of data security and privacy. Despite current legal and ethical standards mandating the anonymization of medical data for research, patients voiced that keeping their data anonymized and their privacy secure remains their top priority and issue of concern. Still, several of these patients admitted that if they were assured that their data would be kept anonymized and would be securely stored with respect to current industry and legal standards, they would be willing to participate in research. While a small number of patients expressed doubts as to whether their healthcare provider (i.e., the National Health Service) can effectively keep patients' health data secure from hackers and data leaks, the majority of patients comprising this interview sample conceded that they had little to no knowledge of how their health data might be stored, kept secure, or circulated beyond their medical provider's institution.

8.3 Lack of knowledge about legal mandates and fears of insurance complications

Many patients also disclosed that they were unsure of the dictates that ethical review boards and legal frameworks impose on researchers working with health data. While all of the U.S. patients interviewed were at least aware of the federal legislation known as the Health Insurance Portability and Accountability Act or HIPPA (if not also other federal statutes such as GINA or relevant state laws), in contrast, U.K. patients, with the exception of those whose profession involves health data-handling, disclosed that they typically unaware of U.K. statutes regarding health data protections to any degree of notable detail. Regardless of whether this ignorance stems from a lack of interest, from trust in the National Health Service to fully comply with the mandates of legal ordinances, or some other reason, both U.K. patients and U.S. patients alike indicated a concern that current legal frameworks are likely too lax in ensuring the protection of patients' ability to access healthcare via private insurance. This was the second most frequently cited concern related to health data-sharing and research participation across the interview corpus. "I am deeply concerned this data will make their way to insurance companies and affect premiums," one patient asserted. In the event of a data breach or a scenario in which data mining allowed health insurance companies to have access to individuals' health data subsequent to sharing their medical data for research purposes, patients questioned whether current law is robust enough to prohibit health insurance companies from obtaining their medical data for purposes of denying them coverage or limiting their access to coverage through higher fees for coverage based on data originally shared for research purposes.

8.4 Understanding other demands for securing consent

Beyond issues of data security, patients consistently related several other factors that would influence their decision to share medical data with a corporate entity for AI and drug development research related to oncology. Most frequently, patients expressed that they would be willing to share their data with companies for these purposes provided their research was explained to them in full and that they agreed with the ethical imperatives of the study and corporation more broadly. In this vein, patients were consistent in insisting that they wanted to know: (1) the research objectives of a potential study, (2) if the study posed any risks or potential for harm. To a slightly less degree patients asserted that they would also want to be informed about where their data would be stored once shared and who it would be handled by, who would own the data once it is shared for research, if their data to kept for future use or circulated for use in other studies, how the study was to be funded and executed, and how the corporate entity manages their profit motives with ethical mandates. Moreover, if provided with all this information, some patients explained that they would then only be willing to share their data if the company designed their research with the imperative to benefit as many cancer patients as possible. For instance, two patients related that if a pharmaceutical company was aiming to conduct research for a drug that would have only a minimal effect on patients' well-being and outcomes such as only be able to "prolong life for two months" based on "the need for profit" then they would not be interested in sharing their health data. "Big Pharma," another patient emphasized, "is difficult to trust." Others noted that they would want to gather more information about how the hypothetical company may or may not be engaged in depriving some patients of necessary treatments. One patient explained that if a company had a history of using patients' data to help create drugs in order to then charge exorbitant prices that placed the drug out of reach for a majority of patients, they would not be willing to share their data to aid a company in their research. Still, two patients conceded that the future prospect of production of generics in this scenario would satisfy them enough to want to share their data. In addition, some patient interlocutors asserted their desire to be updated about the status of the research and its potential outcomes. Likewise, patients wanted to be assured that if researchers handling their data were to find something medically concerning or relevant to their future health status (e.g., a genetic predisposition for a disease) that they would be notified by the research body although some admitted that they were unsure as to how this would be accomplished given de-identification of the data.

8.5 Concerns regarding corporate ethics and the potential for targeted advertising

Moreover, patients insisted that additional regulatory safeguards are needed both in the U.S. and in the U.K. to protect patients participating in research not just from healthcare coverage issues, but also from the potential for corporate surveillance and targeted advertising based on their medical data. Specifically, patients indicated that they believe that sharing their health data with entities beyond their healthcare provider and health insurer could potentially expose them to further and more intrusive corporate surveillance and targeted marketing. Although the inherent profit motives of private corporations admittedly troubled some patients, this factor and the potential of targeted marketing alone did not compel any patient interlocutors to declare that they would refuse to share their medical data based on these factors. Rather, patients related that they would take a "holistic" view of: the company, its research aims, the procedures and mechanisms of the study, and why and how a company might ask participants to transfer ownership of their data and further circulate it beyond the individual study. "Before I share my data," one patient concluded, "I would really need to interrogate the company and its aims."

Critically, patients widely differed in their insistence of how data security and related issues might be pertinent to their decision to participate in research for oncology drug development and AI One U.S.-based patient advocate who primarily works with low-income cancer patients offered an explanation to suggest the variance with which patients stated these issues as relevant matters of concern. She contended that patients' awareness of and inclinations to voice such concerns regarding data security and privacy are contingent upon their health status, resources, and level of education. She explained, "I don't know how much patients know about the extent to which their health data is being shared. I don't think I do either but to the extent that I do know...gosh, I think 'Wow, I didn't know that!' So I don't think most people know...Sometimes with advocates may be higher resourced or have come through [their treatments] and are now stable because in the thick of it I don't hear patients being worried about [issues related to medical data-sharing] during the thick of treatment. Also, we have many clients who are less savvy about the system, and that is, lower resourced here, generally. So I haven't heard a word about it. They are concerned with their personal privacy when it comes to their social security number, their immigration status, et cetera but as to whether they are concerned with their local CVS selling their data out? I don't think they are concerned with that. I think that concern is a higher Maslow level than for instance, 'I'm in treatment and I gotta feed my family.'" In this advocate's view, patients' likelihood to be concerned about the aforementioned issues of data ownership, security, data brokerage, threats to insurance coverage, and targeted corporate advertising necessitated a health status, insurance status, and an educational background that would allow them to consider such issues as sufficiently critical and indeed, the data collected by the author did not seem to dispute this view.

8.6 Genetic data-sharing: fears of discrimination and lack of knowledge and value

A smaller number of patients related they feared that in the event of a health data breach, or of medical data circulation subsequent to a private entity's transference of patient data to health data brokers following research participation, some individuals might be subjected to discrimination or stigma based on their healthcare status, data, or medical history. Patients were particularly concerned with discrimination and corporate surveillance with respect to genetic data. Although patients often insisted that they believed genomics "provides an additional path for predicting the cause of cancer," that it will potentially "improve personalized treatment," and that "generally speaking, they see few negatives to [genomics] research," many related that they remained apprehensive of what social effects the study of such data might entail and communicated fears related to the stigma of medical

DOI: http://dx.doi.org/10.5772/intechopen.92787

genomics. For instance, some held fears of how genetic studies might embolden some researchers to take up "social genomics studies" reminiscent of the twentieth-century eugenics and pseudoscientific approaches to genetics. In further explaining these qualms, patients cited the potential for discrimination related to genetic pre-dispositions, STI or HIV/AIDS status, or mental health histories. As a result, a large portion of patients indicated that as legal protections against such ramifications are, by their estimations, weak or fail to account for contemporary use, patients may demand additional assurances from private entities engaged in health research that if they were to participate in research by sharing their medical data with them, their data would be secured to the highest possible standard and sufficiently de-identified. As one patient explained, "As as it can be de-identified with confidence, then data leaks may be less harmful." Some patients raised other concerns about the current lack of education regarding genomics and cancer patients, corporate actors, and oncologists possess. One patient contended: "I think the field is still early. I am concerned about commercial tests that may not be looking at the same genes and may give different results. Genetic counselors are a must!" Patients possessing these concerns were adamant that genetic data and genomics research needs to be coupled with educational initiatives and expert roles to explain results, consent procedures, and possible harm.

8.7 Issues of financial compensation, benefit-sharing, and medical inclusion

Finally, although most of the patients comprising the interview corpus were willing to share their health data for research without the prospect of financial compensation or benefit-sharing possibilities, approximately 15% of the interviewees (both U.S. and U.K. patients) stressed that these issues would greatly influence their decision to share their health data with a private entity. This issue was particularly important for patients who were currently undergoing treatment. One patient, a mother in her early forties currently undergoing treatment for a rare cancer type, explained her interest in financial compensation and other benefit-sharing as well as how it would affect their decision to participate in private research: "Compensation is nice but I suppose if they can't compensate and then can't use the data, I would rather them be using the data if it's going to be for the greater good and improving medicines and technology. I suppose it would be nice to know what they are working towards. So, in turn, they share: 'This is what we are trying to achieve.' But I sort of assume that if they use your data and have anonymized it by the time they do the study there's really no way of them being able to come back and say, 'This is what we've done with your data.' In a case like with [the pharmaceutical company who makes a drug I need access to in order to attain a higher chance at survival], if they used your data to create a drug and then sell it for a sky-high price that you can't afford, I think that's wrong in a way. Why should they sell it at this sky-high price if they've used this data which has come to them as a free resource? Why is that fair? I suppose I've not really thought it through to that extent when I've given permission [before however] because I just think if this is research, it may possibly help me or help someone else in the future. [So] I probably would still want them to have the data. But maybe there should be other controls to stop them charging the Earth! Just making these drugs and saying, 'these drugs are really amazing but you can't have them because they are ridiculously expensive...We've made these drugs from your data which we have gathered and now we will sell them for 'x' amount.' So yeah I suppose we would want some financial gain if you are going to be passing your information off to these companies...I would want the NHS [National Health Service] or say, Cancer Research UK, or someone like that just to use my data but maybe it is a bit different if you are talking about a big pharmaceutical company that's making billions of dollars or whatever...They can afford to compensate you... and yeah there's generics and I get that. I know that they will come out with generics for [the drug I need] eventually, but that's too late for me. I need it now." This patient interlocutor's explanation of their conditions for medical data-sharing for research participation offers a sense of how patients currently undergoing treatment are conceptualizing the issue of sharing their data and how they wish to benefit in the event of doing so.

In contrast to this patient's understanding of the value of their medical data and sense of how it might be valuable for other actors, many patients expressed puzzlement and apprehension with regard to how their data might hold future and current value. For example, one patient related: "My major concern is that there's not enough knowledge to really benefit [for and as a patient currently undergoing treatment] from shar[ing] this health data [including genetic data, with researchers]. I really wish it could accelerate and that we could use AI to guide the treatments but there's not enough treatments out there to make a massive difference. I hope that it will progress soon...but today I don't really know what you could do with this data that would impact your life in any way." In addition to patients' doubts that participating in research would have a significant impact on the health outcomes of current patients, other patients were confused as to how, in the event of a data breach, their health data information might be of value to others including hackers, government agencies, or corporate entities. "Why would someone want to hack into a researcher's storage system and take my data" and "why would someone want to re-identify my data?," some patients questioned. One patient insisted that this would have no bearing on a decision to participate in research: "But why someone want to do it? I don't really see any reason. So no, it [is not and] wouldn't be a worry for me."

In addition to issues of financial compensation, some patients noted that issues of consent regarding medical data-sharing were of critical importance to influencing how likely they are to share their data with researchers for AI advancement and drug development. As several patients were insistent that medical inclusion of diverse populations in research must be a priority, some asserted that they would be unwilling to share their health data with researchers if they did not make the interrelated issues of patient trust, efficacy, and medical inclusion key to their research. To this end, these patients wanted researchers to prioritize building relationships to recruit diverse populations for their studies, offer educational initiative to help equip potential participants with sufficient knowledge regarding what impacts and effects their participation might result in, and be committed to sharing resources and the benefits of "lower-resourced" populations. Only a demonstration of such commitments could impel these patients to want to share their data for research.

9. Patient-centered approaches to building frameworks of trust and accountability

This section examines patient-centered recommendations and proposals for ensuring patient trust, participation, and safety pertinent to increasing the development and clinical use of AI systems for oncology. Building on cancer patients' concerns, this section highlights three major arenas for cultivating frameworks of trust and accountability crucial to advancing these systems and ushering them into clinical settings. Drawing from the qualitative data produced by this study in addition to the insights of other researchers, these three imperative arenas in need of reinforcement include: Building Knowledge and Redressing Consent and Resource Sharing; Addressing Health Inequities for AI Accountability; and, Promoting and

Establishing Additional Safeguards. Strengthening patient support, understanding, and participation in AI-related oncology drug development requires robust, varied responses to these three interrelated arenas of concern from a multitude of relevant actors. This section provides an overview that attempts to synthesize the attitudes, positions, and actions stakeholders can undertake to broadly ensure accountability, equity, and patient trust and participation with regard to these systems.

9.1 Navigating patient participation and trust: building knowledge, redressing consent, and sharing resources

Educational initiatives remain a critical aspect to earning trust and maintaining accountability within AI-oncology related research endeavors. Establishing truly informed consent requires equipping cancer patients, cancer patient advocates, and oncology care providers with the necessary knowledge to stay informed and alert about how these systems operate, how they are designed and trained, what ramifications might ensue as a result of their implementation. Cancer patient advocates are particularly vocal in stressing the importance of giving patients all necessary information required in order to understand what potential limitations or risks such systems may incur. They further assert the need for a collaborative approach to both building patient knowledge and to assessing how potential harms and complications are to be addressed. They believe that collaboratively produced and executed educational initiatives will foster support among the general patient populace for public and private investments in both AI development as well as for the infrastructural adjustments within their use may necessitate. Advocates and oncologists alike contend that patients often remain ignorant of the options for medical coverage and care available to them, particularly with respect to clinical trials and other forms of research involvement. This lack of education not only comprises one barrier to participating in oncology-related research and drug development studies, but also may furthermore preclude patients from receiving the highest quality of care at their disposal. Additional knowledge regarding research endeavors and their potential benefits may encourage patients, many of whom profess to be open to engaging in research, to participate in AI-driven oncology drug development studies.

Indeed, many cancer patients, including the interlocutors who informed this study, actively assert their desire to learn more about the AI-driven systems that have the potential to considerably impact their treatment from trustworthy sources. Patient advocates reason that given the aforementioned demands on patients as well as the nature of clinical care, more advocates, researchers, and clinicians must be trained in how these systems operate and in how they might affect patients in order to equip them with the necessary expertise for helping patients navigate and assess the potential ramifications that these technologies may have on their treatment. Undeniably, more initiatives need to be established to educate patients in how machine learning-driven systems operate, what their levels of efficacy are, and what greater social effects they might precipitate. Such educational initiatives would serve as a crucial first step in assisting current, former, and future patients in understanding what crucial arenas can be acted upon to ensure that patients receive the quality of care they deserve. These arenas might include, for example, participating in relevant research or reinforcing support for policies that attempt to carve out how issues of liability will enfold in the face of medical error due to AI system usage. As stated earlier, such educational endeavors may hold higher stakes and greater challenges for patients with "limited access to high quality clinical care, limited health literacy, earned mistrust of medical providers, and those individuals who may be exposed to interpersonal and institutional racism and other discrimination in their healthcare encounters" [14].

Nevertheless, it remains important to consider how matters of securing consent and research participation extend far beyond merely bolstering educational initiatives for patients. For instance, too often issues pertaining to refusal of consent and slim participation are framed as the consequence of ingrained beliefs that stem from cultural beliefs rather than as rational stances toward the injustices of biomedical research from beget from the nexus of material inequities and historical oppressions. Against the myopia of cultural determinism, researchers of technology and medicine contend that patients' (un)willingness to participate in research must be appropriately contextualized as complex responses to biomedicine in socially stratified societies. Ruha Benjamin frames such arguments in the following terms: "If we understand trust and distrust not simply as individual or cultural predispositions that are 'held' by some and not by others, but rather as outgrowths of social relationships that are produced through the allocation of material resources and symbolic power, then we see that techniques for cultivating relationships hinge on redistributing and refashioning those, respectively" [18].

Exemplifying the limitations engendered by material inequities, clinical trials frequently fail to recruit people of color and other marginalized people. This fact holds further significance as research conducted by the U.S. Census Bureau predicts that the white population in the U.S. will fall below 50% by 2045. In conducting interview work, it was typical to hear patient advocates and medical professionals bemoan how clinical trials and other research endeavors struggled to recruit "diverse" patient groups for their studies. Beyond educational matters, advocates, clinicians, and cancer nonprofit directors frequently framed the issue of participation as one dominated by cultural inclinations (some groups are like 'x'—'x,' in this case, being a list of static traits or stereotypes of racial groups) rather than as dispositions toward structural inequities. Through cogent research that examines how clinicians' "'ideas about [their patients' 'cultures'] contribute to health disparities," anthropologist Khiara Bridges contends that "cultural stereotypes and beliefs in the way people from certain cultures 'just are' can be dangerous—and just as racist—as racism" [19]. Demonstrably, cultural determinism can result in deleterious health outcomes.

To combat this, Benjamin argues that it is necessary for medical researchers and health professionals to turn "away from a fixation with distrust and towards the problem of institutional trustworthiness" [18]. This logical turn refuses to heap blame, stigma, or tidy labels of ignorance upon marginalized populations whom medical researchers find it difficult to recruit for studies. Instead, it asks researchers to assume a self-reflexive approach to their work and recruitment efforts and compels them to question how their institution, research body, and associates can be accountable to marginalized populations possessing an earned distrust of medical intrusion whom researchers aim to include in medical studies. In advancing the logical turn from a narrow fixation on issues of patient distrust to the broader problem of institutional trustworthiness, health practitioners, tech developers, and medical researchers may begin to fruitfully rectify inequalities rather than reproduce stale, cultural deterministic, and circumlocutory narratives of why "subordinate groups remain elusive to researchers" [19].

Ethicists and researchers similarly stress the need to rethink current regulations for securing consent for biomedical research. They advocate for a shift from the paradigms of one-time consent to frameworks of accountability that attend to participants' evolving concerns and adhere to ongoing commitments of responsible use of participant samples. They argue that as political surroundings, public opinion, the type of information collected, and the application of this data necessarily shifts, researchers must build *responsive* systems of consent. Consent practices, they argue, must not only integrate ongoing assessments of the risks and implications of their research but also frequent monitoring of patient attitudes, beliefs, and perspectives.

Ethicists assert that more needs to be done to guarantee reciprocity or ensure that participants, not just researchers and their affiliated institutions and funding bodies, are also benefiting from the research. This begins with a willingness to address historical injustices that have contributed to the mistrust that certain groups continue to hold with respect to biomedical research. For some, distributing broad benefits in genetics and genomics research involves making research and research instruments publicly available so that they are not tethered to the limited access that often characterizes commercial arrangements. Ethicists also explain that research organizations can engage in capacity-building in which more richly resourced research organizations collaborate and share resources with "lower resourced" organizations and community participants.

As ethicists continue to advocate for benefit-sharing in research through endeavors like capacity-building and commitments to engaging in open source and public domain initiatives, they also advocate for the redressal of the politics[1] of recruitment itself. As anthropologist Cori Hayden argues "scientific knowledge does not simply represent (in the sense of depict) 'nature,' but it also represents"... (in the political sense) the 'social interests' of the people and institutions that have become wrapped up in its production" [21]. Following Hayden's affirmation of the "coproduction" of all scientific endeavors, Benjamin advocates for attending to "informed refusal" as "a necessary corollary to informed consent—one that extends the bioethical parameters of the latter into a broader social field concerned not only with what is right, but also with the political and social rights of those who engage technoscience as research subjects and tissue donors" [18]. Benjamin explains that "the notion of informed consent—although developed to protect the rights and autonomy of individuals to accept or refuse participation in research—implicitly links the transmission of information to the granting of permission; in consequence, "the request to consent can be interpreted as guidance to consent" [18]. Juxtaposing "informed" and "refusal" thereby acts a signal of necessary humility that recalls individuals' right to refuse participation and recognizes a paradigm in which refusal derives from an educated stance.

It is not enough to recognize that educational initiatives have the capacity to contribute to bolstering research endeavors. Rather, scholars of science and technology and medicine stress how "what matters is not only who is in the room and the intentions of those gathered, but also the structures of participation, modes of inclusion, and assumptions about what forms of knowledge and expression are valid and relevant" [18]. One U.S. based patient advocate incisively summarized these issues surrounding recruitment, knowledge-building, and participation.

"A researcher wants their research to be successful so they write their hypothesis and their aims to prove it. If a researcher has a skewed view about a group, I have seen that they write their study skewed that way. When researchers are doing something where they want to get groups in, I think they have to be honest first. A lot of the times the researchers don't look like the community. So you can't walk into the community and not be willing to hear their feelings. It's important for communities of color to be in research. Part of that problem of not knowing how things affect African Americans, Asians, Latinos, and Native Americans is because they are not involved. But they also don't have a reason to trust. So like I said to someone who was trying to conduct a research project, she said, 'Well I don't look like them' and I said, 'Then you say that.' You don't walk in there and pretend that the people looking

[1] Politics, invoked here, does not solely refer to the mechanisms of electoral issues concerning political candidates or parties. Rather, it extends to the "collective social activity"—"public and private, formal and informal, in all human groups, institutions and societies" which affects who gets what, when, and how [20].

at you do not see that you are a white woman. You admit it. 'I don't look like you. I know that. And here's where my heart lies. I want to hear what you are thinking'. Because at least then you look as though you are there for the right reason and you are not looking to skate around the elephant in the room. Because it is about building relationships. You want someone to participate in your study. You know that people of color need to participate and particularly now that they are talking about precision medicine and personalized care. If people of color don't participate in that then what will they know about us? They won't know anything. We will be in the dark age because we are not participating. Although someone came and talked to us and said 'Getting people to participate in clinical trials even in the white community is low. It's lower with people of color.' but there is something that you already know: tell the truth. [laughs] Say, 'I want to do this research.' But I feel like with researchers if it's with people of color that you don't know and that you have your implicit biased conceptions that were passed down or told to you, you don't want to work with those groups. Like 'Oh I don't want to work with that group because they are this.' When actually, you don't know that. When actually you could make a difference and be noticed where others weren't by stepping out and taking that risk because we already know as medicine is moving in this direction of personalized care, that other populations need to be considered. But you gotta be honest and you gotta figure out how to get them involved and getting them involved is sitting down and talking with them. Not saying 'hey I want to do this research I am going to come into your community and I am going to use you and then I am going to disappear.' But making a commitment to come back to the community and share what you learned. When I worked for American Cancer Society and was in San Francisco... I remember Black people [from the Bay View/Hunter's Point neighborhood] talking about how many researchers showed up and came in, did a research study, got their data and took off and never came back. Well that group never wanted to see another researcher, 'all they wanted to do was use us.' You have to change it. And that, to me, means that you are willing to sit there and hear the difficult stuff...if there isn't a hospital, if they have no way of getting the standard things needed, then how do you partner with other people?...So, researchers,...find out what is out there and available. Because there has to be a way to work around [institutional limitations like funding caps]. Saying 'ok you are only going to fund this but I found these other community organizations and clinics, how can we work with them to try to bring the community you are working with back a solution?' Instead of stopping and saying this is too hard and this is why I don't work with this community. You problem solve."

In addition to building patient knowledge concerning: medical technological advancements, research endeavors, the ramifications of technological interventions, science and technology studies scholars, biotechnology researchers, and patient advocates maintain that health inequities must be robustly addressed. With regard to making health technologies inclusive rather than exclusionary, patient advocates advise developers and medical researchers to seek out and collaborate with communities of color and other socially marginalized groups. They encourage conducting research and creating tech that focuses on and addresses the needs of vulnerable groups. A crucial aspect of such a venture, they assert, involves: building relationships and collaborative problem solving with these interlocutors to ensure that needs of these groups (such as basic access to standard treatment options) as well as the analyst's research goals are met. Patient advocates stress that those willing to be pioneering in this regard will be hailed as vanguards and more importantly, are more likely to be recognized by myriad patient groups as *worthy* of trust.

9.2 Addressing and preventing the entrenchment of existing health inequities via AI tools

Amid the excitement for the potential medical insights machine learning and other AI systems might enable stands an increasingly emphatic chorus of experts urging both the developers of these systems and health specialists to ensure that these systems work to mitigate rather than entrench existing healthcare inequities.

Technology experts and critical algorithm studies scholars implore that we evaluate how these AI models—which increasingly manage and organize our lives—are far from neutral or objective tools. Rather, as mathematician Cathy O'Neil asserts, we must soberly weigh how these instruments are demonstrably encoded with human prejudice, misunderstanding, and bias [22]. One reason for this lies in the fact that these systems and the insights they generate are fundamentally reliant on training data sets composed of existing reference data. Conveying the fallibility of the data-driven paradigm within a different sector, in 2018 Amazon reported that the company was forced to discontinue its AI hiring and recruitment system because it discriminated against women applicants. Amazon's recruiting tool relied on resumes submitted to the company over the previous 10 years—the majority of which came from men. Accordingly, these reference data organized the algorithm to give preference to male applicants and to screen out women applicants vis-a-vis subtle cues in their resumes such as experience in a women's organization or education at a women's college [23].

In another example beyond medicine, in 2016, investigative journalists uncovered how predictive criminal risk assessment algorithms—software used by US courts to predict how likely a person is to commit a crime in the future and relay a recommendation for sentencing to a presiding judge—are prejudiced toward people of color as they consistently recommend stronger sentencing for Black and Latinx people [24]. Scholars, among them Ruha Benjamin and Safiya Noble, and investigative journalists such as Julia Angwin continue to scrutinize the ramifications of integrating AI systems across a multitude of disparate realms among them: housing, finance, news media, welfare eligibility, social media platforms, popular search engines, and healthcare. Their research confirms that AI systems possess the capacity to exacerbate existing social inequities.

As the preponderance of data-driven solutions becomes the norm for healthcare specifically, experts demand that we address how these tools can compound existing disparities in healthcare outcomes. One step toward this remediation, researchers assert, involves educating healthcare providers and developers to ensure they sufficiently comprehend how systemic inequities affect individual health. A robust understanding of the causes, consequences, and modes in which health inequities exist not only affords medical specialists and health tech developers a sense of what research and technological solution need to be prioritized to address injustices, but it can also coincide with a self-reflexive method of medical engagement. In other words, knowing how, why, and what health inequities exist, can allow one to approach health interventions with a heightened awareness of the imbrications and the potentially far-reaching implications of their actions and mediations. It would allow one a crucial frame of reference to question how their instruments and actions might be a catalyst for perpetuating social harm. Many argue that this knowledge is a necessary, fundamental, initial step toward remediating health injustice.

Dr. Tina K. Sacks, a medical sociologist who investigates how race and gender impact health outcomes and a proponent of this kind of knowledge building, advocates for a structural approach to understanding health inequities. Sacks asserts: "Although the dominant paradigm in the United States emphasizes individual choice and responsibility, the empirical evidence indicates that our neighborhoods, schools, jobs, and other factors of day-to-day life shape individual and population health" [25]. Similarly, medical historian John Hoberman analyzes how the historical legacy of racialized thinking is reflected in the contemporary U.S. medical establishment by focusing on how physician racism contributes to health disparities. Hoberman's research suggests that medical providers rely on false beliefs rooted in racial essentialism—such as the pernicious myth of so-called Black "hardiness"—to determine diagnosis and treatment for Black patients [25]. In addition to racial and gendered oppression, in the past several decades, researchers have demonstrated that health and well-being strongly correlate with socioeconomic status. Sacks summarizes: "One of the most important systemic inequalities is unequal access to income and wealth, which may lead to poor health behaviors, chronic conditions, and disease" [25].

The findings of the Institute of Medicine's[2] seminal study of the causes and ramifications of pervasive healthcare disparities in the US and the volume of research it prompted, found physician bias, whether conscious or unconscious, to be a crucial factor in the production of disproportionate healthcare outcomes. Subsequent empirical studies suggest that people of color and ethnic minorities, women, and other people who occupy vulnerable social positions are most susceptible to the noxious consequences of bias and stereotyping. Sacks further flags that "numerous studies have documented that healthcare providers are unconsciously or unintentionally biased against members of marginalized groups, which ultimately leads to difference in treatment across multiple domains (i.e., speciality care, pain management, mental health services, etc.)" [25].

Myriad experts assert that it is imperative that we are cognizant and considerate of how social inequities are embedded into the health data upon which AI systems are built. Due to design and optimization constraints, training datasets primarily utilize the health data profiles of those who can afford and have access to long-term, continuous healthcare as opposed to those who have limited access to care, discontinuous care, or fragmented records. Moreover, data gathered via clinical trials have long been known to be unrepresentative of the US population. Clinical trials routinely fail to recruit people of color and other marginalized people. Recently, investigative journalists at ProPublica reported that Black Americans, Native Americans, and other Americans of color are steeply under-represented in clinical trials for cancer drugs—even when the type of cancer disproportionately affects them [26]. This has translated to cancer treatments that are least effective for the population most afflicted by the disease. Critically, people of color continue to have disproportionately higher incidence and mortality rates for kidney, breast, prostate, and other cancers [14]. Likewise, AI tools designed to detect skin cancer have proven less adept at diagnosing skin cancer in Black and brown patients than white patients [5]. While people with fair skin have the highest incidence rates for skin cancer—the most prevalent human malignancy—the mortality rate for people with darker skin such as African Americans is considerably higher. Eric Topol contends that this is especially noteworthy for genomic studies driven by machine learning techniques: "First, people of European Ancestry compose most or all of the subjects in large cohort studies, which means that, second, they are of limited value to most people, as so much of genomics of disease and health is ancestry specific" [5]. Prioritizing health equity would not only result in more robust scientific and medical knowledge, but would also constitute a step toward engendering quality healthcare for all.

[2] Now known as the National Academy of Medicine.

Increasingly, health researchers such as Sacks and Jonathan Metzl propose efforts toward remediating health inequities that center on structural competency. They advocate for well-researched efforts at the institutional level that aim to address the enduring effects of historical oppression. For example, Sacks explains that structural competency involves moving beyond obfuscating framings of racism as a troubled American past or simply an individual failing of "bad" or "uneducated" people. Instead, structural competency demands that we analyze how racism constitutes structural phenomenon embedded and reproduced in US institutions such as medical schools and healthcare settings [25].

Technology developers and data scientists, moreover, must also be involved in building structural competency across the institutions they navigate to produce more robust, just, and effective technological instruments. Data scientist Ben Green affirms that "by developing tools that inform, influence, impact important social or political decisions—who receives a job offer, what news people see, where police patrol—data scientists play an increasingly important role in constructing society" [20]. In consequence, Green argues that it is imperative that data scientists move away from conceptions of technological instruments as simple tools that can "be designed to have good or bad outcomes" and instead recognize how the technologies they are developing "play a vital role in producing the social and political conditions of the human experience" [20]. By this logic, Green asserts that data scientists must also come to recognize themselves as political actors engaged in the "process of negotiating competing perspectives, goals, and values" rather than as neutral researchers merely coding away in their offices [20]. The decisions data scientists make and responsibilities they hold "cannot be reduced to a narrow professional ethics that lacks normative weight and supposes that, with some reflection, data scientists will make the 'right' decisions that lead to 'good technology'" [20]. As "technology embeds politics and shapes social outcomes," a position of neutrality remains an "unachievable goal" Green contends, as first, "it is impossible to engage in science and politics without being influenced by one's background, values, and interests [20]. Second, striving to be neutral is not itself a politically neutral position—it is a fundamentally conservative one" as such a stance functions to maintain a radically inequitable status quo. Correspondingly, Green debunks the logic of the common tech refrain: "'we shouldn't let the perfect be in the enemy of the good'" [20]. Green highlights that data science lacks any theories or coherent discourse "regarding what 'perfect' and 'good' actually entail" and furthermore, "fails to articulate how data science should navigate the relationship" between the two notions; instead, such a claim "takes for granted that technology-centric, incremental reforms is an appropriate strategy for social progress" [20]. Green then points to the example of criminal risk assessment algorithms; "even if they can be designed not to have racial bias," he argues, their deployment can "perpetuate injustice by hindering more systemic reforms of the criminal justice system" [20]. While recognizing that data science is capable of improving society, in Green's assessment, a structurally competent approach demands that algorithmic and data science solutions be "evaluated against alternative reforms as just one of many options rather than evaluated merely against the status quo as the only possible reform" [20]. There should not be a starting presumption that machine learning (or any other type of reform provides an appropriate solution for every problem...data science reforms tend to (implicitly if not explicitly) assert that the precise means by which decisions are made is the only variable worth altering. There may be situations in which this assumption is correct, but it should not be made or accepted lightly, without interrogation and deliberation" [20].

Furthermore, patients and patient advocates recommend cultivating patient and health practitioner education in relation to developments in technology and healthcare as a significant step toward getting patients the right treatment involves informing them of their treatment options and of any potential consequences and side effects. This mandates that medical care providers be sufficiently educated to guide patients and that education materials are deliberately designed to be accessible and easily comprehendible (e.g., offering treatment pamphlets in several languages rather than solely in the dominant language). For patient advocates, these three recommendations are critically imbricated in one another. One patient advocate succinctly questioned: "How am I supposed to educate a patient about a new treatment or drug they won't have access to it?" Experts across the realms of healthcare and technology declare that prioritizing health equity necessitates that we create systems of accountability; educate ourselves on the causes and implications of health inequity; and set our aim ultimately at structural interventions.

9.3 Promoting and establishing additional safeguards

As previously discussed, patients, advocates, and other health professionals are deeply concerned that current legal parameters and regulatory schemes are not robust enough to protect them from the ill effects of potential misuse including health data breaches and medical data-mining. In addition to patients, legal scholars, biomedical researchers, computer scientists, and genetic privacy experts are sounding the call for a legal overhaul of the statutes affording protections based on medical data-sharing and for genetic information, in particular.

Taking the example of genomics and genetics research in a U.S. context, legal experts reason that as genetic information is no longer adequately safeguarded by the protections of HIPAA and GINA, Congress and other legislative bodies may need to pass a broadly applicable, special-purpose genetic privacy law. These researchers also deem it necessary for US policymakers to address the issue of de-identified genetic data. Although legislatures could regulate DNA as personal identifying information in attempt to redress the legal loopholes of genetic genealogy, LawSeq affiliates caution that such a law would not prevent individuals from adding their personal genomes to online databases for ancestry purposes. As a result, Joh and other legal scholars assert that state legislatures and attorneys general can and must act to set up guidelines concerning genetic surveillance and policing by law enforcement agencies while, in addition, Congress and the Federal Trade Commission could address the privacy and security issues of consumer genetic data [27]. Although legal experts do not necessarily advocate for stricter controls on genetic data within biomedical contexts, they do stress the need to regulate the practices of commercial genetic testing companies and data mining firms. Fortunately, many consumer testing companies are invested in preserving the trust of their customers. A few have formed an inter-market privacy coalition, re-committed to strengthening their consent clauses, and released public statements declaring they are opposed to willingly cooperating with law enforcement [28]. Given that it is virtually impossible to ensure anonymity for genetic information, researchers in medicine, law, and computer science also recommend establishing restrictions on how genetic data are stored and repurposed. Some, like Yaniv Erlich, endorse the idea of attaching cryptographic signatures to genetic profiles and using blockchain technology to curb potential abuses. Others advocate for utilizing methods of obfuscation. One of these methods of obfuscation is referred to as "differential privacy" [29]. In this method, noise is introduced to portions of the genetic profile to prevent re-identification and repurposing of the data as well as to control access [29]. Nevertheless, the majority of experts across the fields of law, biomedical science, healthcare, and computer science are unanimous in asserting the urgency for stronger legislative protections.

In addition to supporting more comprehensive regulatory and legal schemes for protecting patients' data, patients also want to know how algorithmic systems for medical usage will be audited for safety. They are further concerned with how regulatory agencies will account for the fact and monitor AI systems for use in oncology context given these systems require regular updates. Will each update be monitored for safe use? How will these bodies guarantee standardization measures for these updates? Who will be responsible for potential instances of malfunction or medical error pertaining to these systems? Patients stressed that legislators, technologists, legal experts, and bioethicists must all be involved in producing answers to these queries and in establishing the necessary auditing agencies to assure enforcement and cooperation.

Still, patients offered yet another crucial safeguard that can be implemented across most university-related research institutes and research-driven corporate enterprises with relative ease: the involvement of patient advocates in overseeing studies. One patient advocate explained: "If I can throw in my two cents, I would encourage companies to involve patients and advocates sooner rather than later. And to set up a patient advisory board sooner rather than later even if they are still in development. Because they are going to give straight up advice and they are going to have knowledge and perspectives that researchers haven't thought of. There's no question they will. Researchers don't know what they don't know when it comes to working with patients. But if you bring them in sooner rather than later, they can learn as they go along." As this patient advocate contends, patients, especially trained advocates, can offer incisive critiques and help guide researchers in reducing the potential for harm, irritating pragmatic issues, and major complications patients might encounter as a result of a study or product. Patient advocates can provide invaluable guidance and intellectual, sociological, and psychological insight into what issues are most pertinent and compelling to patients and how best researchers and research institutions can address their needs and concerns.

10. Conclusion

Researchers assert that AI systems can be understood as constitutive of collective contestations of the political realities, ethical liabilities, and financial viabilities immanent to their social production. Following this logic, studying the patient perceptions of AI and AI-led oncology drug development, listening to patient perspectives, and heeding their concerns constitutes a cooperative entry point to preventing harm, avoiding unnecessary risks, and building networks of public consent and approval.

This chapter examined: patient perceptions of AI-enabled healthcare and present inclination to trust these tools to improve health outcomes; the extent to which they express a desire to be involved in the development of proposed AI systems vis-a-vis data-sharing based on their existing knowledge; the concerns and questions they bear regarding the integration and deployment of these technologies; the recommendations and suggestions they are proposing for ensuring patient trust; and finally, what patient-centered approaches to building frameworks of trust and accountability other researchers of medicine and algorithmic deployment are advancing. While this study found cancer patients hold an openness to participating in research and a general optimism for experimental endeavors related to improving patient outcomes that includes AI-led systems research and use, it also discovered that patients maintain a vast array of concerns that must be addressed to protect patients from a series of potential risks and existing avenues for medical harm and neglect. Specifically, this study discerned that cancer patients are troubled by: a lack of clarity and protections surrounding medical data usage, the potential for emerging technologies to exacerbate existing healthcare inequities, and anemic approaches to resource-sharing, consent procedures, and educational initiatives to bolster research participation and patient trust.

Still, this qualitative study maintains limitations in its scope and aims, its discoveries and discussion. Further research, including quantitative research, may of course aid in parsing out the complexities of understanding cancer patients' varied responses to relevant oncology-specific, technological developments. In particular, this study could be bolstered by additional comparative, cross-cultural research regarding the distinctions between U.S. and U.K. patients and how their contrasting medical care systems may affect their healthcare experiences and impact their positions toward burgeoning medical technologies.

Patient approval and participation are not only imperative to developing and improving AI-systems given the need for vast amounts of patients' medical data but also to ensuring the use and future widespread adoption of these tools which possess the potential to improve patient outcomes. It is crucial to attend to patients' concerns, establish stronger frameworks for ensuring patient trust, and implement accountability infrastructures.

Thanks

I am truly grateful to the patients, their relatives, clinicians, nurses, and non-profit directors and employees who granted me interviews. Thank you for your presence, trust, time and for sharing your experiences, perceptions, and concerns with formidable heaps of honesty and vulnerability.

I also extend my deepest thanks to Geoffroy Dubourg Felonneau for his support, to Belle Taylor for her patience and editing efforts, and to the CCG team for a fruitful year and welcoming environment.

Author details

Roberta Dousa
Cambridge Cancer Genomics, Cambridge, United Kingdom

*Address all correspondence to: bobbie@cancergenomics.co.uk; bdousa17@gmail.com

References

[1] KPMG. PDF. London, U.K.: KPMG International; 2018

[2] Day L, Joshi I, Woods T, Reem M. PDF. London, U.K.: The AHSN Network of the U.K.'s Department of Health and Social Care; 2018

[3] Reddy S, Fox J, Purohit MP. Artificial intelligence-enabled healthcare delivery. Journal of the Royal Society of Medicine. Mar 2018;**112**(1):22-28

[4] Elish MC. The Stakes of Uncertainty: Developing and Integrating Machine Learning in Clinical Care. SSRN. Data & Society Research Institute; 2019. Available from: https://ssrn.com/abstract=3324571

[5] Topol EJ. Deep Medicine: How Artificial Intelligence Can Make Healthcare Human Again. New York: Basic Books; 2019

[6] Elish MC, Hwang T. New York: Data & Society; 2017

[7] Mitchell TM. Machine Learning. New York: McGraw-Hill; 1997

[8] Bucher T. If.... Then: Algorithmic Power and Politics. New York, NY: Oxford University Press; 2018

[9] Mackenzie A. The production of prediction: What does machine learning want? European Journal of Cultural Studies. 2015;**18**(4-5):429-445

[10] What to expect from AI in oncology. Nature Reviews. Clinical Oncology. 2019Jan;**16**(11):655

[11] Begg K, Tavassoli M. Biomarkers towards personalised therapy in cancer. Drug Target Reviews. 2017. Available from: https://www.drugtargetreview.com/article/23631/biomarkers-personalised-therapy-cancer/

[12] Ross C, Swetlitz I. IBM pitched Watson as a revolution in cancer care. It's nowhere close. STAT. 2018. Available from: https://www.statnews.com/2017/09/05/watson-ibm-cancer/

[13] Adamson AS, Welch HG. Op-Ed: Using artificial intelligence to diagnose cancer could mean unnecessary treatments. Los Angeles Times. 2020. Available from: https://www-latimes-com.cdn.ampproject.org/c/s/www.latimes.com/opinion/story/2020-01-12/using-artificial-intelligence-to-diagnose-cancer-could-mean-unnecessary-treatments?_amp=true

[14] Artificial intelligence can entrench disparities—Here's what we must do. The Cancer Letter. 2018. Available from: https://cancerletter.com/articles/20181116_1/

[15] Methany M, Israni S, Ahmed M. PDF. The Journal of the American Medical Association. Washington, D.C.: JAMA; 2019

[16] Elish MC, Monteescu A. PDF. New York: Data & Society; 2017

[17] Myers B. Women and minorities in tech, by the numbers. In: Wired. Conde Nast; 2018. Available from: https://www.wired.com/story/computer-science-graduates-diversity/

[18] Benjamin R. Informed refusal. Science, Technology, & Human Values. 2016;**41**(6):967-990

[19] Benjamin R. Cultura obscura: Race, power, and "culture talk" in the health sciences. American Journal of Law & Medicine. 2017;**43**(2-3):225-238

[20] Green B. PDF. Cambridge, MA; 2019

[21] Hayden CP. When Nature Goes Public: The Making and Unmaking

of Bioprospecting in Mexico. Oxford: Princeton University Press; 2003

[22] ONeil C. Weapons of Math Destruction: How Big Data Increases Inequality and Threatens Democracy. Great Britain: Penguin Books; 2017

[23] Dastin J. Amazon Scraps Secret AI Recruiting Tool that Showed Bias against Women. Thomson Reuters; 2018. Available from: https://www.reuters.com/article/us-amazon-com-jobs-automation-insight/amazon-scraps-secret-ai-recruiting-tool-that-showed-bias-against-women-idUSKCN1MK08G

[24] Angwin J, Larson J, Kirchner L, Mattu S. Machine Bias. ProPublica; 2019. Available from: https://www.propublica.org/article/machine-bias-risk-assessments-in-criminal-sentencing

[25] Sacks TK. Invisible Visits: Black Middle-Class Women in the American Healthcare System. Oxford University Press; 2019

[26] Chen C, Wong R. Black Patients Miss Out On Promising Cancer Drugs. ProPublica; 2019. Available from: https://www.propublica.org/article/black-patients-miss-out-on-promising-cancer-drugs

[27] Joh E. Want to See My Genes? Get a Warrant. The New York Times; 2019. Available from: https://www.nytimes.com/2019/06/11/opinion/police-dna-warrant.html?action=click&module=privacyfooterrecircmodule&pgtype=Article

[28] Gangitano A. DNA testing companies launch new privacy coalition. The Hill. 2019. Available from: https://thehill.com/regulation/lobbying/450124-dna-testing-companies-launch-new-privacy-coalition

[29] Erlich Y, Narayanan A. Routes for breaching and protecting genetic privacy. Nature Reviews. Genetics. 2014;**15**(6):409-421